Anxiety Disorders

YOUR PERSONAL HEALTH SERIES

Anxiety Disorders

EVERYTHING YOU NEED TO KNOW

J. PAUL CALDWELL, MD, CCFP

FIREFLY BOOKS

A FIREFLY BOOK

Published by Firefly Books (U.S.) Inc. 2005

First printing

Publisher Cataloging-in-Publication Data (U.S.)

Caldwell, Paul.
Anxiety disorders : everything you need to know / Paul Caldwell.
[184] p. : ill. ; cm. (Your personal health)
Includes bibliographical references and index.
Summary: Practical health guide to anxiety disorders for both patients and their families, including advice on diagnosis, treatment options and symptoms.
ISBN 1-55297-874-5 (pbk.)
1. Anxiety disorders. 2. Anxiety disorders – Diagnosis. 3. Anxiety disorders – Treatment. I. Title. II. Series.
616.85/223 dc22 RC531.C35 2005

Published in the United States by
Firefly Books (U.S.) Inc.
P.O. Box 1338, Ellicott Station
Buffalo, New York 14205

Printed in Canada

To my wife, Judy,
the best thing that ever happened to me.

Contents

Foreword / 1

Introduction / 3

Chapter One: The Nature of Anxiety / 6

Chapter Two: The Biology of Alarm / 12

Chapter Three: Generalized Anxiety Disorder and Social
                  Anxiety Disorder / 17

Chapter Four: Panic Disorder / 38

Chapter Five: Specific Phobias / 62

Chapter Six: Post Traumatic Stress Disorder / 83

Chapter Seven: Obsessive-Compulsive Disorder / 102

Chapter Eight: Anxiety in Children and Adolescents / 122

Chapter Nine: Treatment for Anxiety Disorders / 134

Chapter Ten: Taking Back a Sense of Control / 151

Table of Drug Names / 160

Glossary / 161

Further Resources / 164

Index / 167

Foreword

Anxiety disorders affect one in four persons at least once in their lifetime. Approximately half of those affected do not seek treatment and suffer significantly in almost every aspect of their lives. The lives of their families are also affected. There is a very significant economic cost to society associated with anxiety disorders, including non-psychiatric medical care, mortality costs, workplace costs and the costs of psychiatric care. The costs associated with anxiety disorders are estimated to be over $42 billion per year in the U.S. alone. The costs of the associated human suffering are incalculable.

Many people seek treatment only after years of suffering. There is still a social stigma related to anxiety disorders, which is, at least in part, due to lack of understanding that these are real illnesses with effective treatments readily available.

This is why I am delighted to introduce this comprehensive, well-written and empathetic book on anxiety disorders. Dr. Caldwell gives us important information in a clear, interesting and easily understood way that will, hopefully, allow people to better understand these illnesses and seek treatment for themselves or encourage friends and family to do so. His use of case studies is particularly effective in bringing these disorders to life for the reader.

Early treatment will improve outcomes tremendously, and diminishing the stigma will allow many people to seek and avail of effective treatments, which will dramatically improve the quality of their lives and decrease the enormous economic burden of these illnesses on society.

Information is powerful, and this excellent book will allow many people to better understand and accept these treatable disorders, thus reducing the stigma and increasing timely access to appropriate treatment. Thank you, Dr. Caldwell.

—Dr. F. G. McNestry, FRCP(C)
Medical Director, Mental Health Services, and Chief of Psychiatry, Peterborough Regional Health Centre; and assistant clinical professor of psychiatry, Queen's University.

Introduction

As a family physician, I am privileged to spend my working days treating illness and trying to relieve suffering and pain. Often, thanks to the efficacy of modern medicine, that's not a difficult task. At my disposal I have antibiotics for infections, analgesics for pain and a vast collection of other drugs and treatments for almost any symptom of physical illness you can imagine. Give me a symptom and I can quickly and adeptly begin to help relieve suffering. On most days, and for most medical difficulties, mine is a very rewarding job.

Sometimes, though, it's just not that simple. With problems such as anxiety disorders, the underlying difficulties that produce pain and suffering are not transparently evident, obvious or accessible. They are much more difficult to conceptualize, and they take a great deal of time and effort to understand. Healing is not a simple process.

Of course, we are all anxious, we all worry, we are all "stressed out." The ability to worry, to anticipate negative consequences or events, is a remarkable human ability. Because it allows us to visualize what might happen in the future, it allows us to begin to prepare for such eventualities. In that sense, anxiety and worry are adaptive and protective; for most of us, anxiety is a good thing—an evolutionary system that makes our lives better.

Unfortunately, for almost a quarter of us, the experience of anxiety is different. Instead of being helpful and accommodating, anxiety becomes intensely uncomfortable and disabling.

Anxiety disorders: Number of cases present in the population	
social anxiety disorder	13.3%
phobia	11%
post traumatic stress disorder	7.8%
generalized anxiety disorder	5%
panic disorder	3.5%
obsessive-compulsive disorder	2.5%

Although we use the same word—anxiety—it is important to understand that the experience is different from the normal in two important dimensions. The experience of abnormal anxiety—the feeling associated with it—is much more intense than that of normal anxiety. Far from being helpful or protecting, abnormal anxiety disrupts the usual activities and delights of life—it disables. The combination of these two qualities produces the extreme suffering and pain seen with these disorders, and prevents the normal enjoyment of life.

That's what this book is about. These problems are difficult to visualize and to understand. It is often impossible to identify their specific causes (why this happens to one particular person at this particular time), and they are very complicated, often occurring with other psychological difficulties. Although they are hard to conceptualize, the pain and disability they produce are every bit as real as those of easily visible physical illnesses. They cannot be "seen" in the same way that a fractured bone might be, but they are not imagined or fabricated. The suffering that they produce is excruciating in its severity and prolonged in its duration, often lasting a lifetime.

The book is organized into the several common patterns of anxiety disorders.

- Generalized anxiety disorder is a pattern of excessive worrying over simple everyday occurrences and events.

- Social anxiety disorder (sometimes called social phobia) is a common problem of anxiety related to your perception of how you are assessed by others in a social environment.
- Panic disorder is a pattern of recurring episodes of extreme acute anxiety (the panic attack) and the changes that these make in your behavior.
- Phobias are severe unreasonable fear reactions to everyday objects or situations.
- Post traumatic stress disorder is a collection of anxiety symptoms related to a previous emotionally damaging event.
- Obsessive-compulsive disorder is a combination of disturbing intrusive thoughts (obsessions) and their responses (compulsions) performed in order to reduce anxiety.
- Anxiety disorders in children have their own particular characteristics.

The definitions of these patterns of anxiety disorders might seem quite finite, but many similar symptoms and experiences are shared among the disorders, and many share other (so called co-morbid) psychological difficulties, such as depression. The specific definitions of these disorders are, of course, quite artificial, but they allow us to begin to understand them as separate entities, even though they are all related within the same family of disorders of anxiety.

The good news is that anxiety disorders usually respond very well to treatment. With understanding and therapy, which may include lifestyle changes, the pain and suffering that they produce can be relieved. Whether you suffer from an anxiety problem or you are concerned about a friend or loved one, this book is designed to begin the process of treatment by giving you the essential information necessary to understand the problems.

Let us begin by examining the enigmatic feeling at the core of the problem—anxiety.

ONE

The Nature of Anxiety

Imagine, after a hard day's work, that you are lying comfortably in bed in your quiet bedroom, waiting for sleep to come. You're feeling relaxed and tired, your eyes are closed, your mind is at ease as you begin the slow, peaceful descent into the pleasant vacuum of sleep. And then, just before you fall asleep, you remember that tomorrow there is a problem situation you must face—perhaps an examination or test at school, perhaps an interview or assessment at work, or perhaps a presentation you must make at a business meeting. Within seconds, everything changes. Your mind is no longer relaxed and calm. Instead, you begin to think about tomorrow's problem—what might happen, how you will react— worrying about the possibilities of negative outcome and the difficult consequences. Your mind has become sharper, more alert and focused as it analyzes the possibilities. As you worry, you lose that peaceful feeling of relaxation and ease; you become more agitated, uncomfortable and distressed. Although you might not be aware of it, your heart rate and blood pressure have risen. Your skin is cooler; your breathing has gone from the slow, deep calm of relaxation to a faster, shallower pattern. Of course, all hope of sleep has vanished—your whole being has been awakened, alerted by the thoughts of tomorrow's problem; sleep is no longer an option.

All of these changes have occurred not because of some external factor in the room (such as a loud noise or an intruder), but rather because you began thinking about tomorrow's problem. It was the simple thought that caused the transformation.

This combination of an uncomfortable distressing feeling and the physical changes of alertness is called anxiety. Anxiety has these two dimensions: an internal feeling of distress, and the physical changes of alertness, of excitation. Anxiety is a diffuse, very unpleasant but vague sense of apprehension, of unease, of intense concern about imminent danger or threat. It is usually associated with physical symptoms such as headache, perspiration, palpitations, tightness in the chest, stomach difficulties, diarrhea and restlessness.

Anxiety is not fear, although it shares many of the same qualities. Fear is also a very unpleasant emotion that can cause an alerting reaction in the body. However, fear is a response to a specific external threatening event, situation or object. Fear is your reaction to danger, to something that could cause you injury or pain; if you are out walking at night and a large dog suddenly jumps out at you, barking and snarling, it's fear that makes your heart skip a beat and focuses your mind. The threat of the injury is external, very real and finite. While drifting off to sleep, on the other hand, the worry about tomorrow's meeting is internal. It has come from your own thought processes; the distress it produces is anxiety. Fear is a response to something external; anxiety comes from within.

Surprise! Anxiety Can Be Good for You

Not all anxiety is bad. The process of anticipating future events, analyzing them and considering your responses can be very helpful, allowing you to carefully examine the various possibilities and make preparations. For example, if you have an exam tomorrow, your mind begins to consider what questions might be asked or what parts of the course will be emphasized. You ask yourself if you are adequately versed in specific aspects of the subject. If not, you may very well get up and continue studying. You consider the possibility of failing the examination and the consequences, which may be distressing to you. Essentially, your mind is exploring all the particulars and possibilities, going over imagined contingencies, thus preparing you for whatever may happen. This process of anticipation is helpful. The anxiety allows you not only to consider the possibilities, but also to focus mentally and physically on the problem.

Anxiety allows you a preview, a preliminary glimpse, of a possible outcome or difficulty. This anticipation is an advantage: your mind has considered the options and your reactions to them. Therefore, a certain degree of anxiety is a good thing, allowing you to learn more easily, to achieve more, to perform better and to quickly adapt.

Anxiety Extremes

For some, however, anxiety is not an advantage. Rather, it becomes extreme and exaggerated in its response, a destructive rather than a helpful force, impairing performance and producing marked emotional distress. Excess anxiety robs the lives of those who suffer from it of peace, strains their relationships with family and friends, and causes significant suffering and unhappiness.

Such abnormal anxiety can take many forms:

- generalized anxiety disorder (GAD), wherein the individual experiences excessive, unresolved worrying over simple life events and challenges
- social anxiety that can cause an individual to be overly troubled by how she or he is perceived by others
- panic that can take the form of sudden, unpredictable bursts of anxiety
- phobias whereby the irrational fear of situations or objects, such as snakes or heights, produces extreme or inappropriate anxiety
- obsessive-compulsive disorder (OCD), a pattern of unwanted thoughts that constantly bombard the mind, producing anxiety that can be relieved only by action.
- post traumatic stress disorder (PTSD), a condition produced by profoundly traumatic events that sometimes produce excessive, lingering anxiety and/or disability

How Many Are Affected?

Across all societies, cultures and continents, these excessive anxiety problems are seen with consistent regularity. These types of extreme, disabling anxiety affect up to 25 percent of the world's population at some time in their lives. Most of these disorders are twice as common in women as in men, and often begin in childhood or early adult life. Although disabling, these disorders might not be apparent to those affected who simply believe (because they have had the symptoms for much of their lives) that "that's just the way I am." Individuals are often quite unaware that they suffer from excess anxiety symptoms that diminish their life experience.

Medical conditions causing anxiety symptoms

Hormonal
- hyper/hypothyroidism
- hypoglycemia (low blood sugar)
- pheochromocytoma (a rare benign tumor of the adrenal gland)

Cardiac
- irregular heart beat
- congestive heart failure
- angina
- high blood pressure
- mitral valve prolapse

Respiratory
- asthma
- chronic obstructive pulmonary disease (COPD)

Others
- vertigo (spinning sensation and dizziness often originating in the inner ear)
- seizures
- migraine (with aura)

Drugs/Chemicals
- alcohol and drug withdrawal
- amphetamines
- caffeine (and caffeine withdrawal)
- street drugs (amphetamines—cannabis, ecstasy)

These disorders are quite persistent, and only rarely disappear on their own. Instead they usually persist throughout life unless treated. Although they can be caused by a medical condition, prescribed medicines or chemicals such as caffeine, they are more often caused by a combination of factors, including a genetic predisposition, individual makeup and life events. Interestingly, people with anxiety disorders often show up at their doctor's office not only complaining about the unpleasant feeling of anxiety; rather, 90 percent of them complain about physical symptoms caused when the body tries to cope with the effects of anxiety. These physical symptoms might include:

- insomnia
- irritable bowel syndrome (and pain, diarrhea)
- chronic fatigue
- fibromyalgia (muscle ache and tiredness)
- recurring or persisting pain (back, neck, abdomen)
- chest pain with or without palpitations (with normal cardiac workup)
- headache (recurring or persisting)
- sweating, flushing
- multiple physical complaints affecting different systems (weakness, dizziness, tiredness, nausea, pain, diarrhea, restlessness, fainting spells, tingling in the extremities) for which no medical explanation can be found

Anxiety disorders are not due to any character flaw or lack of moral fiber. They are not within the individual's ability or volition to control; these are not "your fault," nor are you able to treat these disorders simply by "trying harder." Like diabetes and heart disease, these disorders are medical conditions; there should be no shame or guilt associated with them, any more than there is shame or guilt associated with diabetes or heart disease.

The most important point is that these disorders are very treatable. As we shall see, most will respond favorably to therapies designed for that particular problem. An individual does not have to suffer from anxiety disorders forever. Help is available; it begins with understanding the biology of the anxiety response.

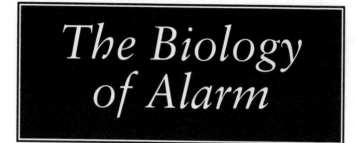

TWO

The Biology of Alarm

We have all had the experience of suddenly feeling frightened, of being alarmed. Suppose, while driving on the highway, the car in front of you unexpectedly swerves, or while quietly attending a meeting, someone asks you to "say a few words." In these situations your body responds quickly and efficiently to help you with the problem. Understanding how this occurs is crucial to understanding anxiety disorders; the response of your body to alarm is very similar to that seen in anxiety states.

Your reaction in these situations is automatic. It doesn't depend on your careful evaluation and consideration of the various options; you just simply "do it." This reflex, this immediacy of reaction, is an important safety feature. You can imagine, throughout human evolution, situations when we simply didn't have time to evaluate all of the ways to protect ourselves from sudden dangers, such as animal attack, natural accidents and other threats. Our ability to react quickly and efficiently is an important, basic, survival skill that we share with other animals. In spite of our huge intellectual capacity, this complex, primal emergency system operates reflexively, independent of our conscious will. While the intricacies of this elaborate system are not yet fully understood, a general understanding of the process explains much of what an individual feels when in the grip of an anxiety disorder.

Mind and Body React as One Unit

In an alarm or danger situation, a sudden change in sensory input usually initiates the process. This change might be visual (such as a large threatening shadow seen out of the corner of the eye), auditory (the barking and growling of a dog), a touch (feeling something while reaching out in a darkened room), or smell (the acrid smell of smoke). This information is relayed to an area within the brain stem called the hypothalamus (part of the limbic system, anatomically located above the roof of the mouth), which is important for regulating our emotions and memories as well as for basic functions like sleeping and eating.

Within seconds, things change. The hypothalamus has connections with other areas in the brain, and these are primed for rapid response in a dangerous or threatening situation. The amygdala (an almond-shaped collection of cells in the brain stem), and the locus ceruleus (a similar group of cells on either side of the base of the brain) immediately begin releasing excitatory chemicals into the brain and general circulation. At the same time, the hypothalamus, through its connections to other parts of the brain, allows you to focus mental energy and concentration on the problem at hand. Rapid thinking and mental processing is facilitated. The chemistry within the brain changes—specifically, the chemicals that carry information between nerve cells (the neurotransmitters) alter in type and concentration, expediting more direct and rapid processing between nerve cells, enabling you to think clearly and quickly. Through its connection to the pituitary gland, the hypothalamus triggers the release of hormones that, in turn, stimulate the adrenal gland (a small gland sitting on top of each kidney) to secrete excitatory hormones called catecholamines. These hormones (norepinephrine and epinephrine [also known as adrenaline]) are quickly secreted into the bloodstream and carried to the rest of the body to prepare it for immediate action. Many physical changes occur because of these hormones; within seconds, the heart rate and blood pressure to rise, thus increasing blood flow from the heart to the muscles and brain. The rate of breathing is increased, allowing better oxygenation of the blood. Blood flow is diverted from the skin to the more essential organs (brain, heart and muscles). Consequently, the skin becomes both cooler and sweaty. Similarly, blood is shunted away from the digestive organs (the digestive function is not a priority in an emergency). The body is on red

Anxiety in the Brain

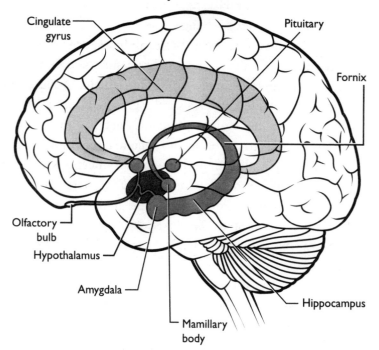

Anatomically, the structures in the brain associated with an anxiety response lie deep within the brain itself.

alert, ready for action. Even the pupil of the eye opens, allowing more light (and thus more visual information) to enter the brain. The adrenals secrete a second group of hormones called corticosteroids, the best known one being cortisol, that affect energy supplies within the body, mobilizing glucose (for the muscles and the brain), decreasing inflammation (in case of injury) and facilitating the biochemical changes needed for a rapid response. In addition, the brain produces morphine-like chemicals called endorphins. These chemicals are pain relievers: in the case of injury, they function to minimize pain so it does not distract from the task at hand. Their presence explains the lack of pain experienced from some injuries and the amazing feats of strength sometimes seen during acute stress.

Effects of the hormones created by alarm

Catecholamines (norepinephrine/epinephrine)
- increase heart rate
- increase blood pressure
- increase blood sugar
- increase cardiac output
- increase generalized sense of awareness and concentration
- increase muscular tension
- decrease blood flow to the gut
- decrease reaction time
- mobilize glucose and free fatty acids to increase metabolism
- cause contraction of smooth muscles in the gastrointestinal and respiratory tracts

Cortisol and Other Glucocorticoids
- increase levels of glucose in the bloodstream (for increased energy)
- break down fat to produce more energy
- decrease inflammation
- facilitate increased muscle power

Endorphins
- decrease pain
- produce euphoria
- decrease sensory awareness (to allow you to focus mentally)

All of these mental and physical changes, occurring automatically in just a few seconds, comprise the body's response to alarm. This response is known as the "fight or flight" response, although, as we shall see, there is another response that becomes important in some phobias—that of fainting. While this ancient, protective mechanism has served us well during our evolution, in anxiety disorders, this response often is no longer protective and helpful. Instead, this cascade of physical and mental changes is inappropriately experienced by the body in response to something that is not, in the true physical sense of the word, threatening. Instead, the anxiety response is initiated by such things as an idea; a concern about a future event; excessive worry; a recurring, disturbing thought; or even difficulty accepting a previous encounter or experience. When these "false" alarms or threats are experienced, the entire complicated process of automatic response takes over, with all of the accompanying physical and mental changes.

It's important to understand that in the alarm reaction there are measurable, predictable physical changes that occur. For example, we can objectively measure the rapid change in body chemistry seen in stressful situations. In one experiment, when interns were asked to present a case at medical rounds, the level of norepinephrine rose seventeen times within just three minutes of the beginning of the presentation. From this example, you can see that these anxiety symptoms are not made up or imagined—not simply "feelings" or impressions—rather, they are the predictable responses to measurable biochemical mental and physical changes. Although the process originated in the brain, the symptoms are not simply "in your head."

Armed with the knowledge of this ancient, powerful reaction complex, we can begin to understand the nature of the disorders produced when this complex reaction—originally helpful and adaptive—becomes exaggerated, extreme and disabling.

THREE

Generalized Anxiety Disorder and Social Anxiety Disorder

"Well, wouldn't you be worried if you had chest pain every day and nobody could find a cause?" Jim asked his doctor. They were in the doctor's examining room, and Jim, a 43-year-old automobile mechanic, was putting his shirt back on. He had just finished another examination—normal again—and had gone over the consultation that his family doctor had recently arranged with a cardiologist. "There must be something wrong—it couldn't possibly be normal."

Over the last year or so, Jim had experienced almost daily, recurring episodes of chest tightness—a squeezing type of pain in his back going around to the front and up into his neck—but no one could find an explanation. Jim was concerned about the pain, and the possibility that he might not be able to continue working or provide for his young family. The fact that no one could find an explanation for the symptoms, in spite of multiple consultations and testing, was of even more concern to Jim. He knew there was "something wrong"—if only the doctors could find it. He was unable to concentrate on even the simplest of jobs at work. The fear that some terrible medical condition was causing his symptoms was never far from his mind. The whole process was so exhausting that sometimes he didn't even have the energy to go to work. Although he was always tired, he usually had trouble getting to sleep, tossing and turning every night. The second he woke up from his troubled sleep every morning he began thinking about the possibility of disability and early death from heart disease or cancer. His days were consumed by worry, and he was very irritable and unable to participate in his family's life. The other night, when his daughter had asked him to help with her math homework, he had been unable to solve the problem, and slammed the book shut in frustration. Immediately he regretted it and apologized—but it was obvious that he was unable to keep his emotions in check. This worried him even more, because he took his responsibilities as a father very seriously.

But now, sitting on the examining table in the doctor's office, he broke down in frustration and anger "I'm falling apart—why can't you find out why?"

Generalized Anxiety Disorder

People such as Jim seem to have symptoms of chronic tension and anxiety most of the time, focused on simple and everyday concerns such as health, family, finances and interpersonal relationships. Since the 1980s, psychiatrists have recognized that this pattern of excessive and uncontrolled worry is common, and can be very debilitating. Generalized anxiety disorder (GAD) has, as its cardinal symptom, excessive chronic worrying about such everyday concerns. Naturally, we all are concerned about our relationships, the growth and development of our family, and our management of money. But in

GAD the worry is different both in quality and in quantity. Although it is often related to the simple everyday events and concerns of life, it is excessive, frequent, uncontrollable and damaging. Apprehension about the future is pervasive, often present from the moment that you get up in the morning until the moment that you try to go to sleep at night. You worry about everything. The distress about the possibilities of danger or some other negative consequence is uncontrollable—you cannot put the problem out of your mind, get on with other business or think about another topic. The worry seems to come back again and again, intruding into thought processes and impairing performance by stealing concentration and focus. Often several problems are the focus of worry, and there is a perception that the cumulative hassles of life are just too many.

To be diagnosed with GAD, such excessive anxiety and uncontrollable worry must be present for more than six months. In addition, persons with generalized anxiety disorder have physical symptoms associated with their chronic worry. Common symptom patterns include:

- Complaints of increased muscle tension (muscles are "tight" or stiff, or people have the feeling of chronic recurring muscle pain because of increased muscle contraction or the inability to relax muscles). People often come to their doctor with headache, neck pain, back pain or stiffness in their muscles.
- A feeling of being restless, "keyed up," agitated, easily startled, fidgety, "antsy" or of being on edge. Inability to relax, settle the mind or enjoy peace.
- Tiredness, exhaustion or fatigue. Chronic worry and anxiety drain the body of resources much needed for other tasks, and

the feeling of being mentally overloaded results. Physical fitness often suffers.

- Poor concentration, with inability or difficulty focusing on a specific topic or problem. A feeling that the mind "goes blank," or that memory is failing (memory depends on concentration), or an inability to manipulate or learn new information normally.

- Irritability. The chronic anxiety produces a pervasive feeling of being unwell and takes away the patience and tolerance needed to accommodate changes in routine, extra demands from interpersonal relationships, and so on. Symptoms of feeling oversensitive, dissatisfied, easily upset or quick tempered, grouchy, or crabby are very common.

- Sleep disturbance. This is extremely common in GAD and usually takes the form of difficulty getting to sleep, waking up repeatedly during the night (with difficulty returning to sleep), unrefreshing sleep, a shortened total sleep time and inefficient sleep (that is, only a small percentage of time in bed is actually spent asleep). Sleep problems contribute greatly to the chronic feeling of fatigue, poor mental concentration and irritability. Sometimes the symptoms of sleep deprivation may be prominent. Excessive tiredness, loss of emotional reserve (with frequent crying or anger), poor performance at work or school, and decreased immunity (recurring infections, such as colds) can be the result.

Because GAD includes both the phenomenon of excessive worry and a combination of physical symptoms, people with this syndrome often go to their doctor's office not because of the symptoms of excessive worry and anxiety but with physical symptoms alone. Although quite distressing and disabling, the excessive worrying is often tolerated by people who believe that this is simply "the way I am." Only 50 percent of individuals with the disorder ever seek treatment, and usually only after they experience symptoms for up to ten years. Of those who do go to their doctor, only about 50 percent are correctly diagnosed. Symptoms—such as insomnia, muscle pain (for example, chest pain, neck pain, chronic back pain), abdominal pain with diarrhea, dizziness, shakiness, restlessness, recurring headaches, shortness of breath, sweating, and palpitations—are often what bring the sufferer to the doctor, and multiple investigations soon follow. The individual does not connect the symptoms of anxiety and worry with the unresolved physical problems. Usually no specific physical abnormalities are found, and, unless the underlying chronic anxiety is diagnosed, these people are treated symptomatically for their physical complaints. The mental anguish (the distress of chronic worry) is not the focus; it's the physical symptoms (caused by the anxiety) that are more prominent. In one study, 80 percent of patients with GAD sought help for their physical complaints and only 20 percent preseated with a psychological problem. Because the physical complaints are a direct result of the chronic anxiety, usually no specific cause for the physical symptom can be found, in spite of multiple investigations and consultations. Sometimes these people are erroneously diagnosed as having chronic fatigue syndrome, chronic ligamentous, disc degenerative back pain, fibromyalgia, migraines, irritable bowel syndrome or any number of other physical ailments.

Who Gets GAD?

Like so many of his generation, Robert had been looking forward to his retirement for years. He had risen through the ranks of employment at the factory where he worked, taking great pride in the fact that he had been the supervisor of the evening shift for the last twelve years. He had been, as the president said at the retirement dinner, someone the company could count on, someone able to handle any problem that might arise.

But since retirement, Robert found that his days were not filled with pleasure and enjoyment. Instead, he seemed to spend much of his time concentrating on the problems of his life and his family. It wasn't that he found himself in the midst of a crisis, but he had three grown daughters with families, and his wife had developed arthritis. It just seemed to him that there were things to worry about every day, from the time he got up until the time he went to bed. He was irritable all the time. He had headaches and complained that he couldn't concentrate. Whatever he tried to do—even if it was something simple, like gardening or reading the newspaper in the morning—he found that his mind kept going over things that might happen. He couldn't seem to put the thoughts out of his head. The same thing happened when he tried to go to sleep at night or even sometimes while he watched television. He felt fatigued and overwhelmed. He was particularly concerned about the possibility that one of his family might be injured while traveling in a car. The possibility of anyone in his extended family taking a long drive would have him worried for days, imagining the anguish and pain of a possible accident. He knew this was not reasonable, but he couldn't help himself. On a couple of occasions one of his daughters had driven on a holiday for several days without Robert's knowledge. When he learned of the trip, he immediately felt guilty—because he hadn't known about it, and thus hadn't worried about it—as if the mere fact of his worrying about an accident would have prevented one.

His family doctor diagnosed Robert's symptoms as GAD, and initiated treatment with counselling and medicine. Within a few weeks, Robert was able to understand the pattern of his abnormal worrying and to begin to enjoy his retirement.

GAD is very common; it affects 5 percent of the population during their lifetime and is twice as common in women as it is in men. Although it often begins at a young age (in one study the median age of onset was twenty-one years), and can be seen in children, it becomes more frequent as we age. In one study, the prevalence (the number of diagnosed cases in the population) was only 2.3 percent of persons aged 18 to 24, but rose to 4.4 percent of persons aged 35 to 44, suggesting that older people worry more and for longer periods than do younger people. GAD is common in seniors—in one study the prevalence was 20 percent, making it one of the commonest anxiety problems of older life. There is a genetic predisposition to the disease. First-degree relatives (parents, children, siblings) are five times more likely to share the diagnosis as the general population. Studies of twins confirm a strong inherited tendency. In identical twins (where the genetics are the same), if one twin is diagnosed with GAD, the chance that the second twin will develop it is 50 percent. However, in nonidentical twins (where genetics are only partially the same), if one twin develops GAD, the chance that the other twin will develop it is only 15 percent. This implies a strong genetic predisposition. GAD has been found to be more common in those who have been previously married (divorced, widowed, long-term relationship) than in those who are currently married, and in those who work at home (including homemakers) rather than those whose employment is elsewhere. Race and income levels were not associated with risk, nor were education, religion or geographic location.

In some people the disorder begins after a life crisis such as the death of a spouse, financial difficulties or the breakup of a relationship. Such events seem to be more common as we age as initiating features for the disorder—being more notable in those whose GAD started later in life. The full-blown syndrome is rare before age twenty-five, and some investigators feel that there are two different patterns: GAD with an earlier age of onset associated with a childhood history of fears, anxiety, chronic social difficulties and a disturbed home environment; and a second pattern of late-onset GAD, often precipitated by a stressful life event.

Why Worry?
At the heart of GAD is the concept of excessive worry. We all worry; we all focus on negative possibilities for the future and "fuss" about these—the possible impact on our lives and the negative consequences. In GAD, however, the nature and particulars of worry are different, and it is these differences that fuel the chronic symptoms.

The *Canadian Oxford Dictionary* defines worry as "to give way to anxiety or unease; to allow one's mind to dwell on difficulty or troubles." The word itself comes from the Old English *wyrgan*, meaning to strangle. A "worry wart" is one who habitually worries unduly. Worrying is an attempt to solve a mental problem that has not yet arisen. To worry about something is not always a bad thing. Normal worrying allows one to consider the possibilities that might occur in the future (particularly negative events) and to prepare for these eventualities. It allows a preview, a "look ahead," to evaluate a possible negative outcome, and to begin the process of deciding what you can or cannot do should such a situation arise. Normal worrying is thus very much an advantage: should a negative consequence actually come about, you will be at least partially prepared. Worrying for most of us is thus the beginning of the process of problem solving. Beginning with the question "what if ...?" you allow your mind to both imagine a negative outcome and to explore the options. This kind of worry is helpful and normal. It gives you a sense of control.

The abnormal worry of GAD begins the same way with the question "what if ...?" but the process of worry seems to be disrupted soon after this. In normal worrying, once the negative consequences are examined and possible reactions and adaptations considered, you are able to move on to other topics and functions. The problem, the worry, has been addressed. It might not be solved but it is manageable. In GAD this is not possible. Rather than functioning normally, the worrying process never seems to lead to a reasonable course of action, leaving the individual with a chronic unresolved and frustrating problem. The worry does not solve anything; it fails to provide any possibility of an acceptable solution. This is why the worry returns again and again, intruding into other mental processes and causing excessive distress.

Not only is the quality or nature of their worrying different, individuals with GAD also seem to have much more to worry about. They have a sensitivity to the relatively mild difficulties of everyday life, believing that "If anything can go wrong it will." They find fuel for worry in almost every encounter and situation. A single problem is not the focus of worry, but many concerns (that are ultimately unresolved) and possibilities fill the day. Such things as children's progress in school, the return on financial investments, the possibility of motor vehicle accidents, being perceived by friends as inadequate or any one of a million possibilities occupy their mind, draining both energy and peace. They have a tendency to view ambiguous or neutral situations as negative, imagining the worst disasters and threats in what others see as innocuous situations. They fear more, worrying that every minor problem will become a full-blown disaster—a phenomenon known as catastrophic thinking. Older sufferers of GAD tend to worry more about health concerns; younger sufferers, although they do worry about their physical well-being, are more likely to worry about their social status and evaluation by others, their job competence and their interpersonal relationships. Interestingly, around the world in different cultures and places, the concerns seem to be quite similar.

Sometimes individuals with GAD, aware that they are "worry warts," even begin to worry about their excessive worrying—a problem that has been called "meta worrying." The worry itself has become a cause for more worrying. In addition, worrying sometimes takes on a magical quality, with the process (and intensity) of worrying by itself having the power to alter events and protect against a negative outcome. It is not uncommon for individuals with GAD to believe that a negative outcome is more likely if they don't consider it and worry sufficiently about it. For example, a mother might believe that the chances of her children being hit by a car on the way to school are much less if she worries about this possibility—that her suffering (through the anguish of her considering the awful event) will somehow protect them.

GAD is usually a chronic condition, with symptoms persisting over a lifetime, often with significant life events causing a worsening of symptoms. Occasionally, in about 20 percent of cases, the disorder will go away on its own.

The Burden of Generalized Anxiety Disorder
Other psychological problems are frequently associated with GAD. In one study, fully 90 percent of GAD patients had

another psychological diagnosis; depression was seen in 62 percent of cases, alcoholism in 38 percent (often an attempt to deal with the chronic anxiety), social phobia in 35 percent and panic disorder in 25 percent. These other psychological problems often compound the diagnosis and management of the disorder, and increase the burden of the problem.

At first glance, it might seem that simply worrying too much might not drastically interfere with life. However, most people with GAD have pervasive and disabling psychological symptoms. Consistently, across many studies, sufferers complain that their lives are much altered by the process of worry, and that they are unable to function. They are mentally preoccupied by the abnormal and unresolving worry and consequent anxiety. In addition, the disruption of their physical well-being (by such things as chronic pain, insomnia and fatigue) severely affects their lives. Because they are unable to focus or concentrate, such simple pleasures as reading, crossword puzzles, even watching a movie or television can be difficult, if not impossible. There is a lack of flexibility and ease in interpersonal relationships; they cannot "let themselves go"; interactions with family are difficult and often unfulfilling. Physical symptoms, so much a part of the syndrome, are present most of the time and detract from their quality of life—not only because of the symptom itself (often chronic pain) but also because of the multiple investigations and consultations that these difficulties usually incur, and the medications (such as painkillers or muscle relaxants) that are often prescribed to deal with these symptoms. Education and employment opportunities are limited, as are possibilities for the enjoyment of life. In addition, as in panic disorder (see Chapter Four), sufferers of GAD often actively try to avoid those situations in which their worry is escalated. Sometimes this avoidance behavior is quite severe. For example, they might refuse to ride in an automobile, fearing an accident. Similarly, they might avoid any social gatherings out of fear that something might go wrong at the function or even that there might be a possible spread of infection with so many people present. They shun attendance at plays and movies (the images or ideas portrayed might expand the possibilities for worry) and, in general, life experiences and enjoyment are severely truncated. Many have developed so-called "safe behaviors"—actions that they believe will decrease the chance of a problem developing—that are sometimes complicated and demanding.

Diagnosis

As with other anxiety disorders, there is no blood test or laboratory work that can prove the diagnosis; rather the syndrome is identified by the symptoms already outlined. It is important to note that excessive anxiety and worry can be produced by many medical problems (such as hyperthyroidism) or by many medicines (such as any stimulant medicine or caffeine). The following screening questions may be helpful in deciding if GAD exists.

- Have you been bothered by feeling worried, tense or anxious most of the time? (90 percent of those with GAD say "yes".)
- Are you frequently tense or irritable and do you have trouble sleeping?
- Do friends or family see you as a "worry wart"?
- Do you worry about things that will not happen or that you cannot change?
- Are you unable to stop your worrying—to put it aside to focus on other tasks?
- Does your worry affect your sleep or your daily activities?

Treatment

Cognitive Behavioral Therapy

Studies have shown that cognitive behavioral therapy is a very effective treatment for GAD. Therapy usually begins with education about the nature of the disorder, the concept of abnormal worry and an understanding of how this kind of chronic worry impacts on daily life. The way an individual thinks, or approaches a potential problem, is crucial to treating GAD. Early identification of the cues of abnormal worrying is important, as is the understanding of the abnormal automatic thoughts (negative) that occur and inflame the worry. This educational aspect is usually supplemented by teaching some form of relaxation therapy to achieve control over the worry and chronic muscular tension that it causes.

An important part of therapy focuses on examining the individual's understanding of the thoughts and beliefs that accompany worry, because these responses are considered to be crucial in solving the problem. For example, in order to put the possibilities into their correct perspective, you are asked to consider "What would be the worst thing that could happen, and how likely would that be?" Examining the underlying assumptions (such as "The world is a very dangerous or unpredictable place") that are often premises for abnormal worry is fundamental to progress. These beliefs or assumptions, often acquired from life experiences, color your interpretation of situations. In addition, controlled exposure to situations that might produce excessive worry is gradually and progressively introduced, along with the teaching of new techniques to handle these situations. This allows you to rehearse the skills that would be important in minimizing the effects of the situations in producing worry. Attention to proper sleep habits (to achieve restorative sleep), the avoidance of stimulants (such as caffeine), regular exercise and attention to substance abuse (such as alcohol) are also emphasized.

Pharmacotherapy
There are a number of drugs that can be used to treat GAD.

• **Antidepressants:** Many studies have shown that this group of drugs is very effective for the treatment of GAD. In addition, because depression is so common in those with GAD, the antidepressants have a dual benefit—treating both the anxiety and chronic worrying, and also the symptoms of depression. Selective serotonin reuptake inhibitors (SSRIs) and serotonin-norepinephrine reuptake inhibitors (SNRIs) have been shown to be effective in many studies, though they may transiently increase the anxiety or tension at the initiation of therapy. Tricyclic antidepressants are also effective, particularly clomipramine and imipramine. Sometimes it is necessary to use a short-acting benzodiazepine (such as clonazepam) to help with sleep difficulty at the beginning of antidepressant therapy. (Details of the various classes and types of drugs can be found in Chapter Nine.)
• **Buspirone:** Buspirone may be effective in the treatment of GAD, particularly the symptoms of worry, tension and irritability. It seems less effective for the physical symptoms (such as chronic pain). Buspirone may take several weeks to take effect. However, many people complain of dizziness when they begin treatment, which may limit its use.
• **Benzodiazepines:** There is no question that benzodiazepines reduce the anxiety and the insomnia of GAD, but the current thinking is that these drugs should not be used as a sole treatment for the syndrome. Although they do help the anxiety

symptoms, they are not effective in treating the depression that is often present in the disorder; in fact, they can make depressive symptoms worse. They are not usually effective in eliminating worry, one of the most important aspects of the disorder. In addition, the development of a tolerance to the drug and of side effects such as dizziness, decreased memory and poor concentration limit their use. In general, they are used for short periods of time at the initiation of treatment and for intermittent specific therapy (for such symptoms as insomnia). Thirty-eight percent of persons with GAD have a substance abuse problem (such as alcohol), and these patients must exercise extra caution with benzodiazepines.

Social Anxiety Disorder (Social Phobia)

As usual, everyone at the gathering was having a good time—
except David. It was the end of the school year, and David
and his classmates were celebrating at a pool party. Some were
swimming, others were laughing and talking beside the pool.
David wasn't very good at parties—he always felt uncomfortable, couldn't seem to relax—and he was very poor at making
small talk. He'd already had a couple of beers to relax and
even now he sat on the edge of the pool by himself, not joining
in, feeling uncomfortable and shy. He just didn't want all of his
friends (especially the girls) seeing how boring and unattractive
he was. He was sure they would all think he was a "jerk."

Alice, one of the girls in his class, noticed David sitting by
the pool and came over to talk to him.

"Why don't you join us David?" she asked.

David could feel himself blush. He was sure Alice would see
it too. He felt hot all over, very uncomfortable, and he began
to sweat. He knew he had to answer her but couldn't look

directly at her. He smiled and said, "Oh, I'm okay here," stammering just a little on the "okay." Alice smiled, and David felt horribly embarrassed, knowing for certain she was laughing at his embarrassment, his shyness. "She must think I'm a complete idiot," he thought. His heart began to pound, he tried to smile back but couldn't. All he could think about was getting out of there, away from the crowd, away from the awful embarrassment of this humiliating experience.

"Well, gotta go now," he blurted out, even though the party had barely begun. Then he quickly left Alice and the party, walking home alone in the warm summer night, cursing his shyness. In his heart, David knew the others were right—he was hopelessly inadequate, hopelessly shy, hopelessly embarrassed.

"They're right," he thought "I am a jerk."

Most of us feel slightly uncomfortable in a crowd, when meeting strangers, when asked to say a few words at a meeting, or in other social gatherings and occasions. This mild sense of unease is quite normal, focusing our energies and mental acumen and helping us prepare for the encounters or interactions. For some (like David), the anxiety is not helpful and can be so intense and severe that the sufferer is unable to function. This condition is known as social anxiety disorder.

In this common disorder, intense anxiety and fear is triggered by social situations in which an individual thinks she or he might be humiliated or embarrassed when evaluated by others. Any situation in which you are exposed to scrutiny can trigger the reaction. Common situations that cause social anxiety can include:

- any social encounter or gathering
- meeting new people

- speaking in public
- making small talk
- asking a question in class
- using public facilities, such as washrooms
- eating in public restaurants

In other words, any situation in which behavior or performance could be evaluated by others.

Social anxiety can be generalized (that is, it is related to most or all social interactions) or it can be precipitated by one or only a few social situations (such as public speaking—so-called performance anxiety). Exposure to or anticipation of the situation produces symptoms such as sweating, stammering, trembling, inability to concentrate, acute loss of self-esteem and a feeling that one will lose control.

Interestingly, blushing is frequently seen in this anxiety disorder—the only one in which blushing is prominent. Some theorize that blushing is a readily visible physical sign of embarrassment or submission, an important physical cue to others that a person is not dominant in a social situation.

All of these symptoms reinforce the fear of appearing foolish, stupid, incompetent, uninteresting or inept in public, and thus reinforce the disorder. There is another difference between normal anxiety in encounters with others and social anxiety. Most of us are uneasy when asked to speak in public, especially if we are unprepared. However, our discomfort is fairly easily overcome and we are able to complete the task—the acute, initial anxiety abates as we speak. In social anxiety disorder, however, thoughts of humiliation are paramount and, as we speak, the anxiety increases concerns about appearing inadequate or incompetent. Our performance weakens as we realize how foolish we must look, and eventually, we are unable to continue.

Global anxiety

Extremes of anxiety are found in all countries and in all societies; the form the anxiety takes is affected and modified by the culture and the setting—examples of such culturally specific anxiety disorders include:

Running amok: *amok* is a Malaysian word meaning "to engage furiously in battle," and refers to an episode of wild, unpredictable and uncontrollable violence, usually resulting in property damage, injury or death, and frequently followed by a period of amnesia.

Koro: a panic-like state seen in Asian males who fear that their sexual organs are retracting into the abdomen and that this relentlessly progressive phenomenon will result in their death. It often relates to an inappropriate sexual indiscretion in the past. Individuals sometimes design complicated devices to prevent the genitals from retracting. Females can fear the retraction of nipples, breasts or labia.

Pa-leng: "fear of the cold" is the literal translation of this Chinese term, whose sufferers exhibit cold hands, an increased heart rate and a morbid fear of the cold. They believe that the balance of yin and yang necessary for health is disturbed, with an excess of yin (the energy-zapping cold) overwhelming the yang (the warm, bright and energetic part of life).

Ataque de nervios: seen in Hispanic Americans, particularly from the Caribbean, this anxiety problem resembles a panic attack but often includes shouting uncontrollably, "speaking in tongues" or breaking into tears. In addition, sleep paralysis, a terrifying phenomenon of waking up after sleep but being unable to move—even to open the eyes—is very common. Sleep paralysis, a phenomenon in which the muscular immobility of REM sleep persists into the waking state, is often associated with the feeling of extreme dread and sometimes by frightening visual hallucinations.

Who Gets Social Anxiety Disorder?

Social anxiety disorder, with a lifetime prevalence of 13.3 percent, is the most common anxiety disorder (and third commonest psychiatric disorder after substance abuse and depression). Usually it begins in adolescence, around the time that young people are expanding their social contacts and learning the more complex processes of social interaction involving those outside the family; for example, members of the opposite sex, teachers, friends and co-workers.

Although the disability can be severe, most sufferers feel that they are simply "shy" and adapt to their "shyness." Their discomfort in social situations is so extreme that it quickly leads to avoidance of those situations that cause the discomfort. This avoidance leads to progressive isolation and demoralization, the belief that they are somehow inadequate, just as they suspected. Consequently, they limit their contact with friends and family, avoiding social interactions, presentations and other situations where they perceive themselves as being inept. If they cannot avoid these occasions completely, they try to limit their exposure within encounters. Dating and interaction with the opposite sex is often severely restricted or completely avoided, and further schooling, occupational training or community work are undertaken only after the likelihood of being exposed to such situations is assessed. This can have profound effects on their future, as young people decide to avoid school and job opportunities because of their perceived inadequacy, or due to the possibility of distressing interactions with others. In one study, nearly half of those with social anxiety disorder were unable to complete high school, and most adjusted their education and occupational training to minimize social contact.

Co-Morbidity

The word *co-morbidity* refers to the association of one abnormality with another. In social anxiety disorder co-morbid psychological problems are common. For example, 40 to 50 percent of sufferers have major depression, increasing the psychological burden. The marked distress experienced by individuals with social anxiety disorder may explain some of the co-morbidity, and the isolation and avoidance often mean that an individual's support network, such as family and friends, is quite limited. The younger the sufferer at the onset of the disorder, the higher the co-morbidity. Alcoholism and drug abuse are also commonly seen, as these agents are used to decrease the "nervousness" and anxiety symptoms. Many individuals are unaware that they have an anxiety problem, simply accepting their "shyness" as part of their personality. Many people participating in substance abuse programs have underlying unrecognized social anxiety disorder as a cause for their substance abuse. Sometimes, the distress becomes unbearable; both suicidal thoughts and attempts are increased in social anxiety disorder.

Treatment

Social anxiety disorder, though often very disabling, is usually effectively treated with a combination of psychological therapy and medicines. Generalized social anxiety disorder (in which symptoms of excess anxiety are precipitated by many different social encounters) is often complicated by the sufferers' belief that what they suffer is not treatable—that it is "just me," normal shyness, or poor self-esteem. Treatment usually includes:

- cognitive behavioral therapy (gaining knowledge about the disorder, setting realistic expectations, eliminating negative thinking about social encounters, etc.)
- relaxation training (learning how to control the physiologic escalation of symptoms such as increased heart rate, sweating, difficulty speaking)
- social training (learning such skills as handling oneself during an introduction or making small talk)
- exposure training (the progressive increase in exposure to situations that may cause anxiety, under supervision, in order to desensitize oneself to the situations and to learn appropriate responses)

- medicines (first-line agents include the selective seratonin reuptake inhibitors [SSRIs], such as fluvoxamine, paroxetine, sertraline or other antidepressants)

Discrete or performance anxiety is usually treated with:

- all of the psychological therapies used above
- medicines (beta blockers such as propranolol may be used as needed; benzodiazepines such as alprazolam or lorazepam are also used)

FOUR

Panic Disorder

The episode took Michelle by surprise, as usual. After all, it had been an uneventful morning—perhaps a bit rushed, trying to get the kids ready for school, but without any great stress or confrontation. She was in the van, with the twins in car seats in the back, when she first felt something was wrong. It was hard to describe, this very early sensation, but there was a vague sense that all was not well, that something bad was going to happen. She felt squeezed, as if the van wasn't big enough and was pressing in on her. Almost immediately she became aware that her heart was going much faster than it should. Just as she sensed this, there was a long pause when her heart didn't seem to be working at all, then a wrenching thud as she had several irregular beats in a row. She caught her breath, wondering if her heart was going to stop altogether. She checked the highway, but the road was clear. There was no cause for concern. The boys were unusually quiet in the back seat. All was quiet. But far from being reassured, Michelle's apprehension worsened; she felt short of breath.

She opened the car window and breathed deeply. She began to feel dizzy, the road in front of her seemed to sway a bit, and that really frightened her, with her precious cargo of children in the back seat. Suddenly, there was a cold sweat breaking out on her forehead. She could hear her breath coming in short gasps as if she was smothering, as if she couldn't get up for air through this oppressive feeling. She had to get off the highway—she was unable to continue driving. With great effort, she found enough strength to pull over to the side of the road and put on her emergency flasher. She knew she was in trouble, deep trouble. She wasn't sure whether it was a heart attack, or a stroke, but knew instinctively that it was very serious. She wondered if she was going to die.

It was then, somewhere in the back of her brain, that she began to recognize she was having another one of her "spells." She'd had several before, not nearly as bad as this one, episodes where suddenly she could no longer function because of symptoms of fear—although she couldn't say exactly why she was afraid.

And then the most disturbing thing happened—Michelle felt that she was no longer in the van, behind the steering wheel, but rather she saw herself outside the van looking back at the scene, as if somehow she had left her body behind and was observing the experience not as Michelle, but as someone separate, an objective observer. She could clearly see herself sitting on the side of the road behind the wheel, inside the van—the way she looked, pale and sweaty, breathing deeply and trembling with fear as she gripped the steering wheel. It was as if she was no longer within herself, as if her spirit had risen up and was somewhere above her, looking back down.

Michelle sat in the van, completely out of control, as the powerful feeling surged through her mind and body. There was no future, there was no past, just this intensely uncomfortable present sense of suffocating fear. She was unable to turn the van off, unable to take her hands from the steering wheel, paralyzed by the sensation of overwhelming alarm, as the indifferent traffic whizzed by.

From the back seat came the question "Mommy, why did we stop?"

After consultation with her doctor and some testing, Michelle's "spells," including this episode, were diagnosed as panic attacks.

The word "panic" is derived from the name of the Greek God of nature, Pan—a mischievous creature who presided over woodlands and meadows, and the animals that lived there. Fashioned from the torso of a man, but with the hind legs, horns, and ears of a goat, he must have been quite menacing when he surprised travelers by jumping out from behind bushes or rocks, standing on his cloven feet. Some were so terrified that they died of fright, the result of suddenly seeing this ugly man-beast appearing before them. This feeling of sudden uncontrollable fear or alarm became known as panic.

We have all experienced the feeling of panic, an intense sensation of fear or alarm. Perhaps, as a student studying for exams, you suddenly realized that the preparation you had done was inadequate. You might have been driving in traffic when another car cut you off and, a few seconds later, you felt a rush of apprehension and alarm when you realized the possible consequences. You might have been out peacefully walking at night, your mind wandering, when you suddenly encountered a barking dog. You might have been walking along a sidewalk with one of your children when they strayed off the path, and you realized that their safety was threatened by vehicles on the nearby road. In all of these experiences you would have felt increased alertness, an acuity of concentration and focus as your mind and body prepared to deal with a situation that needed all your resources. You might have been aware of a quickening of the heartbeat and perhaps felt a sudden intake of breath and a sense of apprehension. These are the sort of normal situations that produce and accompany

A history of the diagnosis of "panic"

Descriptions of panic attacks occur in the writings of ancient Greek physicians, but it was an American Civil War surgeon, Dr. J. M. Da Costa who published an account in 1871 of what he called "irritable heart" occurring in combatants of that gruesome war. He described palpitations, dizziness, sweating and many other symptoms of panic occurring on a regular basis without any known cause. Charles Darwin suffered from panic disorder and his attacks (with resulting agoraphobia) kept him close to home after his famous voyage on HMS *Beagle*, preventing him from traveling again. Sigmund Freud felt that anxiety was the signal of the presence of danger in the unconscious. He described "anxiety attacks" and understood that agoraphobia occurred because of the "recollection of an anxiety attack—what the patient fears is the occurrence of such an attack under the special conditions in which he believes he cannot escape it." In England, during World War I, Dr. T. Lewis, an army surgeon, studied soldiers who developed a peculiar syndrome—Lewis called it "effort syndrome"—with many of the symptoms of panic disorder. The soldiers developed these symptoms during physical exercise or in combat. Lewis noted that it seemed to occur in those soldiers with "constitutional weakness" or in those who were "played out" by stress and exposure. He suspected that blood acidosis, produced by changes in carbon dioxide, or that elevated lactic acid levels, produced by the exercise, might be the causes of such symptoms.

panic. This helpful and useful reaction, that mobilizes and concentrates our mental and physical energy, allows us to channel our physical strength and mental abilities to meet a difficult or dangerous situation.

However, some of us experience a form of panic that differs from normal panic in two major ways:

• It usually has no recognizable cause or trigger.
• It is far more intense and overpowering.

These are important differences. They change panic from a helpful and protective mechanism into a destructive and unpredictable medical problem.

Abnormal panic, such as the panic that Michelle experienced, can occur at any time, without any recognizable cause. This is a key difference—the "panic" that most of us feel the night before an exam or some other stress, such as a public speaking presentation, has a distinct, readily identifiable source. The "panic" is simply a reaction to that stress, an attempt by the body to prepare for it. However, individuals such as Michelle experience a severe form of panic when there is no identifiable cause. Such episodes appear "out of the blue" in situations where there is little or no perceived stress, situations such as sitting quietly reading a book, watching a sitcom on television, or even sleeping. This type of panic is a false alarm, an activation of the panic system of feelings and physical changes without a reasonable cause. There is no known trigger, there is no threat, there is no alarm.

The second important difference is the intensity of both the feelings and physical changes that occur during an episode of abnormal panic. The process of mental and physical focusing that occurs in normal panic is fairly mild. The sensations and physical changes in abnormal panic, however, are severe, and of an intensity that is disabling. These signs and symptoms include increased heart rate, sweating, increased blood pressure and rate of breathing, diarrhea and even fainting.

In addition, the rush of overwhelming and abnormal feelings (such as an intense fear of death, the "out of body" experience that Michelle felt, a feeling of being out of control or "going crazy") are so intense and uncontrollable that concentration and the ability to focus are completely impossible.

This type of panic is disabling—far from helping us to adapt to stresses in our environment, this abnormal panic makes us much less able to be productive and enjoy life. The severely unpleasant attacks occur repeatedly and at random; there seems to be no control over them. Individuals who suffer such episodes of panic soon begin to adjust their lives in an attempt to avoid such experiences and regain control.

Panic Attacks and Panic Disorder

Doctors use the phrase "panic attack" to describe a specific, sudden episode of intense fear or discomfort, as already described. Panic attacks are common—in one study fully 10 percent of individuals reported that they had had at least one. Panic attacks are also experienced as part of other anxiety disorders (such as social anxiety or phobic reactions). Panic attacks can come only once in a person's lifetime or they can come again and again. Recurring, unexpected episodes of panic of this kind are referred to as "panic disorder." In this condition, panic attacks can occur frequently, even several times in a day. Individuals, fearing further episodes, become persistently concerned about the implications, such as "going crazy," or the disruption to their lives and work caused by such random episodes. Panic disorder also includes extreme behavioral changes as individuals strive to avoid places or situations that might trigger the attacks.

Thus, the normal, protective and helpful sense of alarm seen in all of us as a defensive mechanism seems to have, in some of us, been disconnected from any reasonable or apparent cause, and intensified to a degree that makes it almost unrecognizable. The combination of these two features makes panic disorder both mysterious and disabling.

Who Gets Panic Attacks and Panic Disorder?

Using the definitions outlined, studies have shown that from 4 to 6 percent of the population suffer panic attacks, and 4 to 5 percent of the population suffer from panic disorder. Both of these disorders are two to three times more frequent in women than in men. Panic attacks can occur at any age—they have been reported in young children and in seniors, but the mean age of onset is twenty-five years. Some people report that their panic episodes begin around a time when an identifiable increase in stress or anxiety occurs: their panic attacks were initiated or triggered by an identifiable increase in stress caused by such things as interpersonal difficulties or deteriorating health.

Panic disorder has a chronic course that, once established is often (but not always) present for life if left untreated. In one study, 30 to 40 percent of patients were symptom free after five years; 50 percent had symptoms, but these symptoms were not bad enough to affect their lives significantly; and 10 to 20 percent had symptoms significant enough to alter their lives considerably.

Like many other diseases, there is a biological tendency toward panic attacks. This means that some of us, from birth, are predisposed to suffer from panic because we have a biological makeup or constitution that is more susceptible to these episodes. We know from studies on identical twins that if one twin has panic disorder the chance that the other twin will have it is very high—about 88 percent. This is much higher than the incidence of panic disorder in the general population, and it implies that there is some sort of genetic mechanism that predisposes people to having panic disorder. We also know that panic disorder runs in families. In one study, 25 percent of first-degree relatives of individuals with panic disorder had panic attacks—that's at least four times more common than the general population. The understanding is that the tendency to be susceptible to panic attacks may be passed on in the genetic makeup from parent to child.

Description of a Typical Panic Attack

Panic episodes, though they might seem overwhelmingly complex and random to the sufferer, follow a recognized pattern that is remarkably similar from individual to individual. The first panic attack, though it is often associated with some antecedent stress, characteristically begins at a time of rest or decreased vigilance. Thus, the panic episode is unexpected. It often begins with a feeling of nonspecific anxiety, sometimes described as a dread or fear, a feeling that "something awful is about to happen," even a feeling of impending death. Often there is an awareness of your heartbeat—it might seems faster than usual or more irregular. There could be a pounding of the heartbeat "in the ears," or a disturbing feeling that the mechanism of heartbeat is dreadfully wrong when extra beats occur. The chest often feels tight and breathing is difficult—resulting in the need to take deep breaths and a feeling of smothering, that one is not getting enough breath, not enough oxygen. Other symptoms include:

- a feeling of choking or coughing—that the throat or upper airway is tightening and "closing off"
- feeling that clothes are too tight and must be loosened
- feeling that windows must be opened in order to get more air
- a cold sweat on the face and hands
- feeling either too hot or too cold
- a disturbing numbness and tingling in the hands and feet or around the mouth
- a visible trembling or shaking of the hands and head, making it impossible to do fine movements, or even to hold a glass of water, or use a telephone

What to do during a panic attack

1. Slow down and control your breathing. Rapid breathing creates many of the changes that you feel during a panic episode.
2. Visualize the progression of symptoms during a panic episode (one thing usually leads to another, for example, increased heart rate leads to palpitations). Try to stop the progression by isolating one event from another.
3. Get to a safe place—where you can lie still or sit down—where you can feel comfortable. This often means getting away from crowds and strangers.
4. Realize that the attack, though it might be uncomfortable, is usually not associated with any risk of harm to you, and that it is finite—lasting only a few minutes; you will soon be better.
5. Tell a friend what is happening so he or she can help you and be a focus for you.
6. Use relaxation techniques to help you focus.

Prevention

Practice relaxation techniques daily. Success in handling panic attacks often comes by having practiced a relaxation technique that you can use at the beginning of any panic episode.

- feelings of abdominal pain, nausea or a fullness in the abdomen; as are both vomiting and diarrhea
- dizziness, the feeling of being lightheaded or about to faint, which contributes to the sense of alarm
- stammering
- loss of concentration
- paralysis

Most upsetting, there is often a feeling, in addition to the sense of dread, that somehow "this is not real," that "it's not really happening." Sometimes individuals feel that they are not in their own body, but are somehow outside the body looking back on it objectively. All these symptoms are accompanied by an overwhelming fear of dying, of "going crazy," or of losing control; they usually appear very quickly, and progress so rapidly that within only a few minutes many of the above symptoms and signs are present. Loss of consciousness can be seen in up to 20 percent of attacks. Attacks often last twenty to thirty minutes, rarely more than an hour, though they can recur several times over a day. Symptoms may disappear quickly or gradually, leaving individuals shaken and exhausted, overcome by the mysterious power of the episode. Usually, the hours and days after the attack are filled with concern about the cause of the episode, and the possibility of future attacks.

Understandably, many patients with their first attack will quickly go to the emergency department or some other medical facility, focusing on the physical aspects of the attack. They are convinced, from the intensity of their experience, that there must be "something wrong" in their body, something life threatening, such as a heart attack or stroke. This disconnect often leads to protracted medical testing that can delay the true diagnosis. In one study, the average time between the first panic attack and the correct diagnosis was ten years.

Some patients, convinced that they are losing control over their mind, chose to suffer in silence. They are afraid that the experience would be unbelievable if described to a friend or spouse, and they try to deal with the problem themselves. They worry that they may be going insane, and they prefer to keep their own counsel, often changing their behavior in an attempt to prevent further attacks.

What Happens During a Panic Attack?

There is no doubt in the minds of individuals who suffer from panic episodes and who understand the pattern of symptom production that there must be some powerful physical phenomenon occurring to cause these drastic changes. It feels as if there should be some overwhelming surge of excitatory chemicals released in the bloodstream to effect such marked changes throughout the body. Unfortunately, scientists have not been able to clearly identify such a simple explanation. Current understanding is that panic episodes occur in those who are predisposed to panic because some trigger initiates a cascade of biochemical and physical changes, not all of which have been clearly identified.

For many sufferers, one of the most difficult aspects is trying to understand the cause of the unexpected onset. Occasionally, a trigger factor can be identified. For example, studies show that exercise can induce panic episodes. It is thought that the buildup of lactic acid in the bloodstream, as well as the increased heart and respiratory rate caused by exercise can "prime the pump" of a panic episode. The phases of the menstrual cycle can be a nonspecific cause of panic, with episodes being more common just before a period begins. Also, it is known (through laboratory experiments) that elevated levels of carbon dioxide in the air we inhale can bring on a panic attack. How the mechanism works is not completely clear, but it is thought to relate to the increasing respiratory rate that takes place when the body tries to rid itself of the excess carbon dioxide. This mechanism seems to apply where there is poor ventilation, such as a crowded elevator, a hot and stuffy room, or obstruction to normal air flow by a scarf, or by an upper respiratory infection or cold. In these situations, a panic attack is more likely. Caffeine can bring on panic episodes, even in those who have never suffered an episode. Interestingly, our sensitivity to caffeine increases as we age. This sometimes means that panic attacks appear unexpectedly when we simply maintain a moderate caffeine intake. In other words, as we age, the same dose of caffeine will affect us differently.

How to help someone who is having a panic attack

1. Be gentle and calm. Although it might be frustrating for you, the situation is very difficult for your friend, who needs you to be calm so that she can focus.
2. Take her to a safe place, ideally to a spot where she can lie or sit down, out of the sight of strangers. Be sure it is a safe place.
3. Focus on breathing; try to help her slow her breathing down, to once again obtain control. If necessary, breathe with her.
4. Touch her. Physical contact (holding a hand, arm around the shoulder, etc.) is quite helpful and reassuring—the touch helps to ground her to reality.
5. Reassure her that the attack is finite and will end soon, and will not do her any harm.
6. Use imagery for relaxation. For example, "imagine you are on a warm beach out in the sun, relaxing …"
7. If you know your friend's relaxation technique, use it with her.

Prevention

Practicing relaxation techniques before a panic attack occurs is the most effective way of dealing with the symptoms once the attack begins. Helping individuals learn relaxation techniques, practicing the techniques on a regular basis and then performing these techniques together during an attack has proven to be the best way to help someone having a panic attack.

However, trigger factors such as these are often not present and indeed many times there don't seem to be any events or situations that would initiate the cascade—in fact, exactly the opposite. The attacks occur when alertness and vigilance are at a minimum and when everything seems calm and relaxed. One interesting theory postulates that those who suffer panic attacks are more aware of their body's sensations than those who do not and that, in conditions of low external stimulation (such as quiet reading, resting or watching television), individuals with panic attacks "sense" minor changes in their bodies' functions (such as heart rate or breathing pattern) that might not be noticeable during activity or exercise. This heightened awareness of bodily sensations is then overemphasized and associated with a feeling of alarm or fear, which in turn initi-

ates the panic attack. We have all had the experience of notic-
ing our heart rate when we are resting quietly. In most of us
this observation imparts no sense of concern or alarm, but this
might not be the case, the theory suggests, in those who suffer
from panic disorder.

Chemical Changes During a Panic Attack

For years, scientists have attempted to identify chemical
changes within the body during a panic attack. Some studies
have shown an increased amount of the breakdown products
of norepinephrine, or adrenaline, the hormone secreted by the
adrenal cortex in response to a "fight or flight" situation. Although
it is well known that this hormone can produce panic-like
symptoms, it has not been found to be universally present in
increased amounts during panic episodes. However, in some
studies, the hormone has been seen in increased quantities particularly in the fluid surrounding the brain. Norepinephrine,
when injected into the bloodstream, does produce many of the
effects of panic, such as increased heart rate and blood pressure, and does produce a feeling of increased alertness.
However, most studies have shown that during a panic attack,
levels of the hormone in the blood do not change.

A second biochemical change that has been studied is that
of hyperventilation. Hyperventilation is the term used to
describe breathing at an abnormally rapid rate, and it is a
symptom commonly seen in panic episodes. In this situation
more carbon dioxide than usual is eliminated from the body
(because of the increased respiratory rate) and the loss of this
carbon dioxide changes the acidity of the blood. This, in turn,
changes the availability of chemicals such as phosphate and
calcium in the cells of the body and the brain. Because altered
levels of these chemicals can produce such symptoms by chang-

ing the way muscles contract, these changes could be responsible for some of the numbness and tingling seen in panic episodes, as well as the shaking and trembling. In addition, low carbon dioxide levels in the blood can produce narrowing of the blood vessels. Positron emission tomography (a technique whereby the uptake of blood is measured in areas of the brain) has shown that constriction of the blood vessels in the brain is commonly seen in panic attacks. This could be the mechanism that is responsible for producing such symptoms as dizziness, fainting and a feeling of doom.

Because so many of the symptoms of panic involve brain function (such as the feeling of impending death, of "going crazy" or of disassociation) several investigators have looked at the levels of neurotransmitters within the brain. Neurotransmitters are chemical messengers whose function is to carry information from one brain cell to another. An increase in concentration or facilitation of these chemicals might cause increased transmission of information, and thus produce symptoms of hyperalertness. Unfortunately, there has been no consistent finding of alteration of these chemicals during a panic attack.

Thus, in spite of years of research, there has been no single biological or chemical mechanism found to adequately explain all of the complex changes that occur in panic. The understanding now is that this ancient, protective alarm system of panic—that works so well when an identifiable threat is present—is somehow malfunctioning, as though there has been a "false" alarm. Not only is this alarm false but the response to it is also much more intense and overreactive than the normal, protective true alarm reaction would be. It is as if the mind and body have overshot the mark, producing such a severe, overexaggerated response that, far from protecting us from danger, is in itself a danger.

How Panic Attacks Affect Your Life

Any individual who suffers from panic attacks will agree that they are among the most unpleasant experiences possible. Not only can you not predict them but, during them, you lose control completely. You are unable to function, to do even simple things such as caring for children or driving the car. You may lose consciousness or fall, have uncontrollable shaking and trembling, be unable to speak or communicate, and are otherwise completely disabled. Such symptoms are extremely embarrassing, almost as frightening to those who observe them as they are to you. You would do anything to avoid them.

In an attempt to prevent such disastrous episodes, many sufferers restrict their activities and experiences. Agoraphobia, the fear of places that might trigger an attack or where an attack might be difficult, is one of the commonest restrictions (see page 67). Agoraphobia is a conditioned response, an association between the attacks and a particular place; as a result, individuals commonly restrict their movements and travel. This is one of the commonest coping mechanisms, as individuals try to arrange their environments so that they are "safer," and the chances of having an episode are lessened.

In addition to avoidance, there are other methods used to reduce the chance of having a panic attack. Any sensation that could produce feelings or sensations commonly seen at the beginning of a panic attack must be avoided. For example, a rise in heart rate is normal during exercise, but individuals with panic disorder will sometimes refrain from exercise completely, fearing that the normal increased heart rate response might trigger a panic attack, or even that the sensation of a rising heart rate, so similar to that experienced during panic, is too terrifying to risk. Similarly, they might steer clear of dancing, sexual relations, walking quickly or getting angry, fearing that the sensation of an increased heart rate present in all these circumstances "feels like" the beginning of a panic attack, and might initiate one. Equally, sitting in a hot stuffy room might produce the same sensation of shortness of breath that they have experienced as one of the initial symptoms of a panic episode. Thus, sufferers studiously avoid these situations, refusing to take a shower or bath with the doors and windows closed or drive in the car with the windows up. Drinking coffee or eating chocolate, with the mild stimulation that the caffeine in these products produces, also reminds them of the panic attack and is, therefore, eliminated from the diet. Anything that might begin to frighten them, such as a horror movie or an amusement ride is assiduously shunned. All these situations might be evaded or

Nocturnal panic

You would think that people who suffer from panic would be allowed some much-needed rest while asleep. Unfortunately, the factors that cause panic attacks do not "sleep," even though the brain is resting. Thus it is quite common to have episodes of panic at night, awakening you from sleep. Such episodes tend to occur earlier in the night, during the phase of sleep between Stage II ("light" sleep) and Stage III ("deep" sleep). In the transition between these stages of sleep, breathing and heart rates normally become erratic—it is theorized that the irregular breathing rate might change carbon dioxide levels in the blood, triggering a panic attack, even in sleep. At one clinic, 25 percent of individuals with panic disorder reported at least one nocturnal panic attack. Commonly, the first symptom upon wakening is a feeling of dread or impending doom, quickly followed by the usual physical signs, such as a racing heart, shortness of breath and sweating. It is important to differentiate these nocturnal panic attacks from other sleep disruptions, such as sleep apnea—a condition in which the upper airway intermittently closes, preventing air movement, and resulting in repeated awakenings, often accompanied by a loud gasping for breath and a sense of alarm. The phenomenon of nocturnal panic simply means that our brains are still capable of processing information and reacting, even though our bodies are asleep. This type of panic attack responds to the same treatment as panic episodes experienced during the day.

in someway restricted—not only because they produce sensations similar to those experienced during a panic attack, but also in the fear that they may precipitate an attack.

Many individuals, in an attempt to minimize the effect of the panic episode once initiated, have so-called "safety behaviors" that they use on a regular basis. For example, some will not travel without their anxiolytic medicine, or will take along supplemental oxygen, or a fan to keep them cool. These safety behaviors are used to not only prevent an episode but also, should one occur, to minimize its effects and/or duration.

Sometimes, disabling panic attacks continue to occur, despite such attempts to prevent them. As a result, individuals often become severely affected, restricting their activities and social interactions accordingly. The attacks become a dominant force in their lives. They live in fear of the panic episodes, afraid of even the possibility of an attack, really afraid of fear itself. This can render the sufferer a recluse, afraid to leave his house for fear of inducing an episode. Diets and activities can be severely restricted, without any resulting effect on the repeated attacks. Sufferers are unable to work, unable to sleep (for even in sleep panic attacks can occur) and/or unable to participate in family life. Many are so demoralized that they consider suicide—in one study 20 percent of those with severe panic symptoms had attempted suicide. If you have considered suicide as a solution, contact your doctor immediately to begin to get treatment and relief.

Other Causes of Panic Symptoms

It is possible to suffer panic attacks, completely identical to those already described, from a wide range of causes that are both identifiable and treatable. Thus, in order to correctly diagnose and treat the symptoms, it is necessary to have a careful medical evaluation to rule out these other causes. In addition, many substances, chemicals and illnesses can aggravate panic attacks and panic disorder, causing the episodes to occur more frequently or with greater intensity. Thus it is also important to carefully review these possibilities with a physician.

Medical Causes
As you can see from the table below, many medical conditions can produce panic episodes. For example, hyperthyroidism (a condition in which the thyroid produces excess levels of thyroxine, the thyroid hormone) can produce symptoms of increased heart rate, sweating, headaches or dizziness. A benign tumor of the adrenal gland, called a pheochromocytoma, causes intermittent increased secretion of norepinephrine, and this syndrome may cause panic attacks indistinguishable from those described above. Hypertension, congestive heart failure or even a heart attack may produce many of the symptoms of panic episodes, such as a constricting feeling in the chest, a sense of irregular or rapid heart beat, and shortness of breath. Therefore, careful evaluation by a physician, including appropriate laboratory tests, is necessary to diagnose these medical causes of panic.

Some Medical Conditions That May Cause Panic Attacks

Disease	Symptoms
Cardiovascular disease	High blood pressure
	Cardiac arrhythmias (irregularity of heartbeat)
	Mitral valve prolapse
	Congestive heart failure
	Angina
Lung diseases	Emphysema
	Chronic bronchitis
	Asthma (Acute)
Endocrine diseases	Hyperthyroidism
	Diabetes
	Hypoglycemia
	Pheochromocytoma (tumor of the adrenal gland)
Neurological diseases	Meniere's Disease (vertigo)
	Migraine
	Multiple Sclerosis
	Transient ischemic attack

Chemical Causes

As well as medical causes, a large number of chemicals, both prescription and otherwise, can produce panic-like symptoms. For example:

• When used in even small amounts, caffeine can produce the symptoms of panic in those sensitive to its effects.

• Many over-the-counter cough and cold preparations contain antihistamines and other decongestants.

• Some antidepressants, high blood pressure medicines, even medicines used to stop smoking can produce panic-like symptoms.

• Prescription tranquilizers, sleeping pills or sedatives can produce panic-like symptoms when they are decreased or discontinued.

• Alcohol is a sedative, with the effect of decreasing brain function when it is being used. As the chemical is being cleared from the body, particularly after sustained use, it can produce a sense of hyperalertness or arousal with panic-like symptoms.

• In a similar manner, painkillers, antidepressants, over-the-counter sleep aids, and other medicines can produce panic-like symptoms as they are withdrawn from the body.

The diagnosis of panic disorder is made only after a careful history and physical examination, and elimination of chemicals and substances that may be producing the symptoms.

Laboratory Agents Used to Produce Panic

To study a phenomenon such as panic disorder in a scientific manner, researchers have attempted to produce the attacks in a laboratory setting, in order to identify triggers and evaluate the body's changes during the attacks. A wide variety of agents have been studied, and these studies offer information that helps us to understand the episodes.

After observing that panic episodes were more common in some people after exercise, and that individuals prone to panic attacks produce more lactic acid during exercise than others, scientists tried to produce panic disorder by simply giving lactic acid intravenously. Lactic acid—a chemical normally produced when muscles exercise, particularly during aerobics—is well known to trigger panic attacks in those who are susceptible. However, when lactic acid is given intravenously in a laboratory setting, it seems to produce panic attacks only in those individuals who are predisposed to panic. That is, you cannot produce a panic attack in someone who is not predisposed. This is probably the explanation for the commonly observed association of exercise with panic attacks.

Another chemical studied was caffeine, with similar results. Although it is possible to produce panic attacks in almost anyone if the caffeine level injected intravenously is very high, using levels that would be seen in the diet (for example, up to five to ten cups of coffee a day) seems to produce panic attacks mostly in those who are predisposed. Many sufferers have identified that even small amounts of caffeine can increase the frequency of their attacks, and so avoid caffeine.

Because hyperventilation (unusually deep or rapid breathing) is a common sign of panic disorder, tests have been done that focus on the level of carbon dioxide inhaled. Researchers wondered if an increased level of carbon dioxide in inhaled air might trigger a panic attack. In normal circumstances, the carbon dioxide level in inhaled air is very low. In a series of experiments, scientists increased the percentage of carbon dioxide in the ambient air without telling the subjects being studied. Once again, scientists found that increasing the percentage of carbon dioxide in the inhaled air could trigger a panic episode, but usually only in those who were predisposed—which probably explains the increased incidence of panic attacks in situations where inhaled air is "stale," hot or confined.

A wide variety of medicines and other chemicals have been used to study panic, including neurotransmitters (serotonin, the neurotransmitter important in depression), acetylcholine (another neurotransmitter important in emotional control within the brain) and others. Unfortunately there have been no consistent reports identifying these as triggers.

Thus, there has been no single chemical that has offered us an adequate explanation as to why panic attacks occur in some people and not in others.

Co-Morbidity

The word *co-morbidity* refers to the association of one abnormality with another. Researchers have found that many individuals who suffer from panic disorder also have other psychological problems associated with, and sometimes as a result of, the panic episode. It is important to identify these problems in order to direct treatment.

- **Depression:** With its feelings of hopelessness, loss of enjoyment of life, and sadness, depression is one of the commonest problems associated with panic disorder. In some studies, depression is seen in up to 60 percent of those with severe panic disorder. Though the depression might be secondary to the devastating effects of recurring panic attacks, the association is important because depression can severely affect your outlook and prognosis. The identification and subsequent treatment of depression substantially improves quality of life.

- **Substance abuse:** Alcohol and other substance abuse is commonly seen with panic disorder, in up to 40 percent of individuals with severe symptoms of panic. It is thought that the use of alcohol (and other substances) is an attempt to relieve the symptoms, decrease the frequency of attack and make life more bearable.
- **Obsessive-compulsive disorder:** OCD (see Chapter Seven) is seen in about 10 percent of those with severe panic disorder. Many obsessive-compulsive thoughts and behaviors are an attempt to decrease the frequency of attacks or to minimize the effects of an attack. Agoraphobic behaviour is often quite obsessive, because driven by the fear of further panic, individuals focus on the specific particulars of places and situations.

How Can We Understand Panic Disorder?

As we have seen, there is neither a single, simple explanation for the phenomenon of panic attacks and panic disorder nor is there a single biological mechanism or chemical that can explain everything. However, there is certainly some biological (genetic or familial) tendency toward the problem, and we do know that the onset of panic attacks is often triggered by some sort of stress (although some time can elapse between the stress and the first episode).

The understanding now is that the genetic or familial tendency, the vulnerability or susceptibility, is the most important factor and that this lies dormant, as a predisposition only, not evident or active until some form of physical or mental stress causes the full development of the disorder. Many people cannot identify a specific stress present when they begin to have the problem—it just seems to start on its own. However, the disorder can be triggered by a physical stress.

Sometimes a physical "fright" such as a surgical operation, a pneumonia or a heart attack is the stressor that precipitates the attacks. In one study 24 percent of women with panic disorder had their first episode within months of the delivery of their first child. Other investigators feel that the psychological makeup of the individual suffering the panic attacks is of more importance than a single event or stress. Studies have shown that individuals who suffer from panic difficulties often have early experiences with unpredictability in their life, with resulting low self-esteem and low perceptions of being able to control their life. In addition, such individuals often come from families where their parents focused anxiety on medical problems, such as chronic illnesses, or implied that many symptoms commonly seen in childhood were dangerous and unpredictable. Although none of these factors in and of themselves might cause the disorder, the combination of several of them in a individual who is biological predisposed to panic might very well produce the disabling attacks.

Treatment

The good news is that the following combination of treatment options is very effective for most individuals:

- Cognitive behavioral therapy using a combination of education and understanding to explain what's happening and progressively increasing exposure to the panic trigger to desensitize individuals and give them a sense of control. This is very effective.

- Pharmacological treatment is often used in combination with cognitive behavioral therapy. Antidepressants (such as SSRIs) are the usual first choices. These drugs may have to be used for some time before adequate control is reached, and often they are used in doses higher than those used in the treatment of depression.

F I V E

Specific Phobias

The day was perfect for a picnic. It was spring, and the woods
were coming alive with green. Ellen—a wide-eyed and happy
four-year-old—and her family had chosen to eat their lunch
at a picnic table beside the lake, sparkling in the sun. They
unloaded the lunch basket and food from the trunk of the
car, and Ellen ran ahead with joy. Excited at the prospect of
playing at the edge of the water, Ellen reached the picnic table
first, carrying her bottle of juice. Suddenly, she began to
scream. She dropped the juice that she was about to put on the
table and backed up slowly, shrieking loudly, as if she had been
hurt. Her mother rushed ahead to see what was wrong, but
when she got to Ellen she could not comfort her. Ellen couldn't
speak, but continued to scream, her face red and congested,
eyes wide open, her body rigid. After several seconds, and
while still crying, Ellen pointed at the table though she still
couldn't speak. Ellen's mother looked at the table, but couldn't
see anything that might have upset the child. Then she noticed
there was a spider—the type called "daddy longlegs"—on the
near end of the table. The spider was immobile, its long thin
legs lifting its body off the table. Ellen's mother could see
nothing else that was wrong with the table—and didn't understand what was happening to her daughter. She was able to
comfort Ellen a little bit, holding her close, and asking her
"What's wrong, Ellen?" Ellen seemed to quieten down but was

still looking fearfully at the table. Then the spider began to move—running across the top of the table. Ellen began screaming again, pointing at the spider. It was then that Ellen's mother understood—it was the spider that had caused such a frightful reaction in her daughter. Turning quickly, Ellen's mother swept the spider from the top of the table in one motion, then showed her daughter the empty tabletop. Ellen began to settle down, looking apprehensively at the tabletop, at the bench seats and on the ground around her.

Eventually, after several minutes, the family was able to calm Ellen, but she would not sit at the table and refused to eat. They wondered where this severe and unreasonable fear of spiders had come from—they were unaware of any previous experience with spiders that might have caused Ellen to react in such a remarkably abnormal way. Finally, they were able to calm her enough so that she would eat some lunch—but she still refused to sit at the table, preferring to eat standing up, holding onto her mother's side. The picnic had been ruined.

Phobias are severe, persistent and unreasonable fears of an object, situation or activity. They are extremely common in our society, present in 11 percent of the general population. The Greek word *phobos* means fear, terror or flight, and was also the name of a Greek warrior-god who was so fierce in battle that he inspired panic and surrender in his enemies. The first medical use of the word was in a description of one of the symptoms of rabies—hydrophobia, an aversion to water. In phobia, exposure to the feared object or situation produces an acute and severe anxiety reaction, a feeling so uncomfortable that, even though sufferers realize that the intensity of the fear is unrealistic, inappropriate in the situation and unjustified, they will do anything to remove themselves from the situation or object.

The Difference between Fear and Phobia

Fear, the unpleasant feeling of apprehension caused by exposure to or anticipation of danger, is a normal protective emotion that allows us to anticipate what might happen and prepare for the possible outcomes. In this way, fear is an adaptive, helpful and appropriate emotional response, functioning to protect us in a situation that we perceive as being threatening.

Phobia differs from fear in two ways. A phobia is a severe, overwhelming fear—the intensity of feeling is so excessive that it does not protect but rather completely disables, and a phobia is both unreasonable and irrational. However, even though the sufferer knows that the fear is unjustified, it cannot be controlled but persists and recurs at every exposure to the phobic stimulus.

How Phobias Affect Us

There are three parts to the phenomenon of phobia:

- a subjective response (the feeling of anxiety)
- the physical changes that this produces
- the resulting change in behavior (avoidance)

At the core of any phobia is an irrational and morbid fear, a very powerful subjective feeling varying from an acute sense of unease to sheer terror. This feeling occurs repeatedly on exposure to the phobic stimulus. Needless to say, this intense anxiety is uncomfortable and distressing, so severe as to be intolerable. It is not only the physical presence of the threatening object or situation that can cause this reaction; sometimes, just a mental image or even a word can trigger a response.

Physical changes are produced by this sudden anxiety reaction (the severe sense of fear). Heart rate and blood pressure increase, sweating appears and the breathing rate increases. The sympathetic hormones epinephrine and norepinephrine are secreted in excess. As in other anxiety states, there is increased blood flow to the muscle, and brain. In some phobias (those relating to blood, injury or injections) there is a second phase of physical changes, with a drop in blood pressure and heart rate. On each exposure to the phobic stimulus the sympathetic hormones are secreted very quickly. Not only do these hormones produce physical changes, but also change the way a person thinks in the situation. As a result of the combination of the irrational sense of dread or apprehension and the physical feelings that the phobia invokes, an individual will often describe these emotions as, "it's as though I'm going to die," "I'm losing control," or "I'm overwhelmed."

Because the experience of a phobia is so intolerably unpleasant, individuals soon begin to adjust their lives to avoid encountering the phobic stimulus. Sometimes this avoidance behavior is very simple (for example, those with a snake phobia will avoid walking in the woods where snakes are found). But, often it results in more drastic behavior that severely limits their quality of life, such as the agoraphobic who refuses to leave the house. Untreated, phobias usually last for life and can be disruptive and debilitating. Most specific phobias are very amenable to treatment without medications.

Phobia or Aversion?
An aversion is a profound dislike of a certain sensation, such as a sound, touch, taste or smell. For example, the sound of chalk scraping on a blackboard, the hairy feel of peach skin, the irritation of wool fibers (from a sweater or a blanket), or certain tastes and smells may produce an intense reaction of discomfort and unease. There is no fear or anxiety felt during

exposure to aversions—though there might be a very uncomfortable feeling with shivering down the spine and the perception that your hair is standing on end. In phobia, a severe irrational fear is the most powerful feeling.

Types of Specific Phobias
Animal Phobia
An abnormal fear of snakes, spiders, dogs, bats, mice or rats, or "bugs" is the most common phobia worldwide, occurring in 7 percent of the population, and is three times more common in women than men. Within this group, snakes and spiders are the most common triggers for a phobic reaction. Animal phobias frequently begin at an early age (they are often seen in very young children) and usually, but not always, the severity declines with age. Although some individuals fear injury from the animal, such as being bitten or attacked, most are simply overwhelmed by the unbearable possibility of proximity to a creature that is revolting, slimy, scaly or otherwise perceived as being disgusting. The fear is not of the animal itself, but rather of the vague but intolerable possibility of events that might happen upon encountering it—such as contact with the "hairy" legs of a spider or the "scaly" snake, or the unpredictability and rapidity of movement of such animals as bats and mice.

The fear of contamination or disease is also seen as part of this phobia. The intensity of the fear reaction is often marked by an extremely unpleasant subjective feeling of terror and loss of control. Although the phobic stimulus can be fairly easily avoided, some individuals go to great lengths to prevent possible contact, such as rarely leaving the house or going for a walk, for fear that they might encounter "insects." Many sufferers perceive these phobias not as "disorders," but as idiosyncrasies; not illnesses but simply behavioral quirks.

Common types of phobias

- animal: the largest group; abnormal fear of snakes, spiders, bats, rats or mice, dogs, bugs
- agoraphobia—the fear of open spaces or places where escape might be difficult, such as movie theaters, supermarkets, shopping malls
- claustrophobia—the fear of confined spaces, such as tunnels, cellars, or elevators
- nature, the environment: acrophobia—the abnormal fear of heights, storms or thunder, wind or water
- blood/injury/injection: the abnormal fear of having blood taken, seeing skin cut or other injury, or having an injection
- social phobia: also known as social anxiety disorder—the abnormal fear of scrutiny or humiliation by poor performance in social gatherings, public speaking or eating out in public. This can be either generalized (all social encounters) or specific (so-called performance anxiety) and is discussed in more detail in Chapter Three.

Situational Phobia

Agoraphobia (from the Greek word *agora*, meaning market), is an abnormal fear of public or open spaces, in which a panic attack might occur or in which, should such an attack occur, escape would be difficult or embarrassing. It is the most common situational phobia manifesting itself as a fear of such things as:

- entering stores, malls, theaters, restaurants and other public places
- being in crowded or congested places
- standing in a line
- traveling in buses, trains or airplanes
- leaving home alone

The fear can apply both to crowded areas, such a marketplace or movie theater, or to wide open spaces, such as an empty stadium. It is not the place itself that is so frightening to the sufferer but rather the possibility that the place might trigger an overwhelming panic or anxiety attack that would be extremely embarrassing or humiliating, or for which help would not be readily available. Having an easily available exit is critical—individuals look at a situation, assess the chance that they might have a panic or anxiety attack, and then evaluate how easy (or difficult) it would be to stop the attack by leaving the situation or by obtaining help. If there are many people around (such as in a crowded restaurant) humiliation and embarrassment are anticipated fears, should an acute anxiety attack occur. In a wide-open space (such as a flat country road) the fear that no one would be available to help them in the event of a disabling anxiety attack produces the phobic response.

Agoraphobia can occur with panic disorder (see Chapter Four), or alone. It is common—occurring in 4 percent of the population. The anticipation of an anxiety attack is so distressing that those with this phobia change the way they behave—they adjust their lives in an attempt to avoid the situations or places that might trigger an attack. Often, this avoidance behavior significantly affects their quality of life. Individuals spend their lives in "safe" environments, those in which they perceive the risk of an anxiety attack as low; avoiding activities that could produce symptoms that are even remotely similar to those of panic. Thus, many severe agoraphobics are confined to their homes, refusing to travel outside (especially alone). They refuse to shop for groceries, eat in restaurants, attend social functions—such as parties, school meetings and weddings; they avoid physical activities, such as brisk walking, hiking, sexual relations or running up flights of stairs for fear that any of these activities will produce some of the subjective feelings of early panic. Many engage in "safety behaviors," activities or thoughts that make them feel more secure or protected, such as traveling only with a companion, carrying a lucky charm or bottle of medicine, smelling salts or antacids. Not only are life experiences dramatically limited, but contact with family and friends can be severely restricted and distorted. Families often try to accommodate the severe anticipation of anxiety attacks by adjusting their own plans, thus limiting their own experiences and perpetuating the problem.

Claustrophobia (the Latin word *claustro* means closed or locked) is the fear of enclosed, restrictive or confined spaces. It is another common situational phobia, in which individuals experience extreme anxiety in such situations as:

• being in tunnels and cellars
• riding elevators
• sitting in rooms without windows
• traveling on subways
• taking showers
• standing in a line
• sitting in a hairdresser's chair under a dryer
• entering a small toilet stall

All such situations and places can trigger an anxiety attack. Claustrophobia occurs in 2 to 5 percent of the population, and people with this phobia naturally try to avoid situations that they perceive as being likely to trigger an episode. Avoiding confined spaces is difficult in our modern society and complicates life for many claustrophobics. For example, individuals will drive miles out of their way to avoid a tunnel, or might be unable to function if a business meeting is held in a small, windowless meeting room. The fear is not of the room or the tunnel, but rather of the intolerable sense of being trapped, restricted, enclosed—or that free exit is prevented or impaired. A fear of suffocation, of not having enough air to breathe, or a restriction of breathing itself is often mentioned, and the claustrophobic cannot be convinced that there is enough oxygen available. The symptoms of claustrophobia are often quickly relieved by leaving the enclosed space.

Phobias of Nature and Environment
Heights
Acrophobia, the fear of heights, refers to an irrational and overwhelming fear of the possibility of falling, even when safety is assured. Interestingly, the fear of falling is not the primary concern, it is the height itself. This phobia can be severely disabling—especially in our modern multilevel society—because sufferers avoid:

- stairways, elevators, escalators
- high-rise buildings
- windows
- balconies
- ladders
- bridges
- hiking, walking or even driving in hilly countryside

Storms
Fear of thunder and lightning or other types of storm (astraphobia), is another common phobia, in which extreme anxiety is felt in the presence of these natural phenomena. Sometimes this phobia can be so severe that sufferers follow weather reports obsessively and adjust their plans (so as to be inside in a protected space) in the event of any threat of rain.

Water
Hydro or water phobia usually originates in early childhood, with symptoms of extreme anxiety relating not only to swim-

ming or water immersion, but also surrounding bathing or showering. It is surprisingly common, occurring in 5 percent of children under age twelve. This phobia usually (but not always) dissipates by adulthood as children are exposed to water by such things as swimming lessons, water play and the unthreatening nature of bathing. If the phobia persists into adult life, it can lead to the avoidance of swimming (or any water-related activity), or even regular bathing and showering.

Dental Phobia

Most people do not enjoy a visit to the dentist, but see the minor discomfort and inconvenience being justified by the health and dental benefits. Between 5 and 10 percent of the population has a phobia of dentistry, with severe debilitating episodes of anxiety experienced in the dental office, or on anticipation of having dental work done. Many with this phobia (but not all) can identify previous, specific painful or uncomfortable dental work as the "cause" of their phobia. Avoidance leads to poor oral health, dental disease and loss of teeth. These problems can result in a change in appearance and social acceptability, leading to poor self-esteem, embarrassment, and restricted social and family contacts. Interestingly, for some sufferers, pain was not the significant triggering factor but rather the encounter with the dentist, who was seen as impersonal, uncaring, disinterested, cold, or not appreciative of the patient's distress and pain. Sometimes a fear of choking, or extreme distress when foreign objects (such as dental instruments) are put in the mouth, complicates this phobia.

Atypical Specific Phobias

While not as common, it is theoretically possible to have a phobia of *any* object or situation. The most common phobias (as already outlined) comprise more than 90 percent of phobias, but some uncommon phobias include:

- **Disease phobia** (an unrealistic fear of situations that could expose an individual to disease) leads to avoidance of such environments as restaurants, public places and public washrooms.
- **Choking phobia** (a fear of choking to death) can be the result of a single experience of severe choking, or of witnessing such an experience in others. As a safeguard, sufferers eat only soft foods, liquids and easily swallowed

All choked up?

Have you ever developed a "lump" in your throat—the disturbing sensation that you couldn't swallow or speak properly? The medical term for this phenomenon is *globus hystericus*—a malfunction of the small circular muscles of the pharynx (throat) that commonly occurs in emotional states, such as sadness, grief, or even anger and is frequently seen in panic disorder and other anxiety disorders. The symptom was first described by Hippocrates in menopausal women. At the time, it was believed that the *hyster* (uterus) was a floating organ that moved freely within a woman's body—*globus* resulted when the organ rose to the base of the neck causing choking—as if a ball or globe (*globus*) was stuck in the throat. Because the symptom was caused by the moving uterus it was called *globus hystericus*.

We now understand that the symptom is caused by the constriction of the small muscles in the throat responsible for swallowing. Although this muscle constriction might result from any irritation, such as reflux of acid from the stomach, it is most commonly caused by an intense emotional experience that could be as innocent as hearing the national anthem played before an important hockey game. Although it is commonly temporary and of no significance, it can be very severe, with the perceived difficulty in swallowing leading to marked weight loss, avoidance of social situations (especially eating) and preoccupation with the problem. In one study, it was the seventh most common complaint in one ear, nose and throat clinic. The symptoms usually respond to treatment of the underlying anxiety problem.

foods. A choking feeling is often seen as an anxiety symptom in other anxiety disorders.

- **Vomiting phobia** (a fear of vomiting or of the embarrassment associated with it, or witnessing it in others).
- **Flight phobia**, (the abnormal fear of flying), is often classified with agoraphobia or claustrophobia. Individuals avoid flying because they fear the consequences of either being in the enclosed space of an airplane, or of crashing. Although accidents do happen, statistics show that if people could die only in airplane crashes, the average person would live to be one million years old.
- **A phobia of dolls, costume or masks.** These phobias, commonly seen in children, produce acute feelings of anxiety and panic associated with the "force" or "power" hidden behind the external façade.

Blood, Injury or Injection Phobia

At age 15, Marty was no longer a boy, but rather a big and strong young man. He was captain of his hockey team, played soccer and basketball, and prided himself on his stamina, his "toughness."

But he didn't feel tough today—far from it. Marty was scared. Today was the day the public health nurses came to his high school to give immunizations—a booster injection in the arm that everyone had to have. Others in his class were joking about it, but Marty had a marked sense of unease all morning. The class was called down to the school gymnasium, and then one by one they went through the doors to receive the injection. Marty watched his classmates come out after the shot; some were swaggering, but one boy looked pale and his face was taut. Then it was Marty's turn—he walked into the big room and saw the nurse ready to greet him, syringe loaded.

He could smell the sweet alcohol antiseptic, feel his heart pounding, his breath coming rapidly. He knew he had no choice—he had to have the shot—so he rolled up his sleeve, hoping that he could just get through it. The nurse turned to him, uncapped the needle and swabbed his arm with the alcohol. He felt dizzy, the room started to spin, and, even before she could give him the shot, he fell backward, striking his head on the gymnasium floor. The next thing he remembered was the nurse calling his name, kneeling beside him on the floor, shaking him. He felt awful—dizzy, sweaty, disoriented, and unable to concentrate or work out in his mind what had happened. Slowly, he came back to his senses. He was embarrassed, frightened and ashamed—all at the same time. The worst thing was—he hadn't even received the injection!

In this common phobia, occurring in up to 4.5 percent of the population, acute overwhelming anxiety is brought on by the sight of blood, any physical injury (either witnessed or experienced), or by receiving an injection or any other invasive medical procedure; for example, having blood drawn. Most of us have a feeling of apprehension, alertness, and mild distress at the sight of blood or injury. However, in this phobia the reaction is extremely pronounced and can be very disabling. Individuals often refuse to have medical examinations of any sort (including regular checkups), immunizations or regular blood testing. Such avoidance can result in the neglect of proper treatment for serious medical problems.

In addition, individuals avoid movies and plays (where blood and injury could be shown), and are unable to function when they or others, including children, are injured. Some sufferers will avoid visits to the hospital, sporting events and television shows, even reading about any activity or situation

Coping with needle phobia

Almost 10 percent of the population has a marked aversion to needles, experiencing extreme distress associated with the taking of blood or similar procedures, sometimes leading to fainting. Effective treatment is available; like other phobias, needle phobia responds to exposure therapy—gradually increasing medically supervised exposure to blood, needles and visual images of injury. Ask your doctor. Here are some helpful suggestions:

- Lying down, with your legs elevated, decreases the chances of fainting during procedures involving needles.
- Repeatedly tensing and relaxing the muscles in the body (particularly the arms and legs) helps to prevent fainting.
- Becoming aroused (for example, by imagining something that makes you angry) raises the heart rate and thus helps to prevent fainting.
- Decreasing the pain of the needle stick (by using local anaesthetic, available in a patch to be put on before the needle injection or drawing of blood) also helps.
- Sedation (for example, with a short-acting benzodiazepine) decreases the anxiety. It may be used before medical testing or injections.
- If blood phobia is preventing necessary medical treatment (for example, preventing adequate care of diabetes because of fear of needles) it can usually be treated by several short courses of desensitization therapy.

where they might be exposed to images of physical injury, wounding or blood.

Often present at a fairly young age, the dreaded anxiety will direct individuals to avoid certain occupations, such as nursing, teaching, or laboratory work where these triggers and situations might occur. Women might avoid pregnancy and child rearing. Men suffer from the feeling that they are "inferior" because they cannot function at the sight of even the smallest amount of blood. Typically, it is their reaction to the stimulus itself that is the problem. Individuals fear that they will faint on exposure to the stimulus, producing an embarrassing reaction. When present, this blood/injury or injection phobia is usually the only phobia (that is, it is not associated with the fear of heights or small animals). Most individuals with this phobia are unable to explain the disability, believing that they are simply "oddballs" and that the problem is all "in the mind."

Not "Fight" or "Flight" but "Faint"
With this phobia, although the severe irrational fear is the same as in specific phobias, the body's physical response is markedly different, with fainting being quite common. As in the other phobias, individuals exposed to blood or injury have, initially, the same generalized sympathetic reaction: increasing heart rate, increasing blood pressure, and a change in blood flow. In blood/injection/injury phobia, however, this initial reaction is soon followed by a dramatic drop in heart rate and blood pressure that is caused by an opening of the blood vessels in large muscles. This produces sweating, pallor, nausea, ringing in the ears, dizziness and, as blood flow to the brain is decreased, fainting in up to 80 percent of those exposed to the phobic trigger. The individual can become both unresponsive and unaware of his or her surroundings, and is, therefore, at

Is fainting protective?

In spite of the disability that blood injury phobia seems to produce, there may be an evolutionary advantage to the reaction. In some animals (such as the African antelope), when chased by a predator (such as a lion), the initial physical response is the typical flight reaction—with increased heart rate and blood pressure. However, if the antelope is cornered, and escape is impossible, the animal will stop running and lie still, as if feigning death. This has the advantage that sometimes the predator is no longer interested in the prey—as if the immobile animal is not perceived to be alive, and thus less appealing. In addition, the antelope's heart rate and blood pressure fall. This may be protective; low heart rate and blood pressure might reduce blood loss if injury actually occurred. Thus, in humans, the blood/injection/injury phobia may be an evolutionary remnant actually protecting us from physical harm.

risk of falling. Some seizure-like activity might be seen. Sometimes individuals are unconscious for several minutes. This type of phobia usually begins in childhood and usually lasts throughout an individual's lifetime. There is a clear genetic pattern, with the phobia being much more common in first-degree relatives.

Where Do Phobias Come From?

Genetics

It is very clear, from the studies of twins, that a biological, genetic tendency to develop phobias exists within families. For example, relatives of patients with social phobia are three times more likely to develop the condition than are those without such a family history. Similarly, in a study of blood/injection/injury phobics, 61 percent had a first-degree relation with the same problem. In other types of phobias this tendency is not nearly so noticeable—only 31 percent of individuals with a specific phobia of spiders or snakes had a first-degree relative with the same fear.

Previous Negative Experience

A previous painful or frightening experience seems to be a significant factor in some phobias. For example, in dental phobia, more than 90 percent of individuals can identify a previous severely unpleasant encounter. However, in other specific phobias (such as spiders or snakes) only 10 percent of individuals can identify a former negative experience. Some researchers have suggested that, particularly for those phobias that first appear in childhood, the original encounter or experience might not be remembered; it may have occurred before memory was even possible. Most of us have no memory before the age of three or four years—the experiences that we had in those early infant years may never be recalled. However, it is speculated that the emotional component of the experience (that is, the pain or the frightening or threatening anxiety response) may have registered and remained in our brain.

Vicarious or "Secondhand" Experience

Some researchers suggest that in a situation where an individual witnesses others reacting in a frightened or threatened manner—to such things as snakes and spiders—the witness would "learn" to have the same emotional response. Even hearing about negative consequences can produce this reaction. For example, in India, where poisonous snakes can hide in long grass, children are told from a very young age to avoid the tall grass, coupling the anxiety of an anticipated negative experience with the grass itself, which for some might result in a phobia of the grass.

A Conditioned Reflex

Russian physiologist Ivan Pavlov showed by experimentation with dogs that the secretion of saliva could be stimulated not only by food, but also by the sound of a bell when it was rung in association with the presentation of food. He also showed that, eventually, the sound of the bell alone would produce salivation, a phenomenon he called a conditioned, or learned, physiologic response or reflex. Some specific phobias could be conditioned reflexes, in that physiologic changes occur with the presentation of an innocent cue (like the bell for Pavlov's dog). For example, a previous exposure to storms might be associated with another, forgotten, unpleasant experience (such as being cold, wet or otherwise uncomfortable). The original experience is forgotten, but the storm produces the emotional and physical response.

Evolutionary or Prepared Learning

During our evolution, many phobias have related to situations or objects that would be a threat to humans, especially young developing humans. Such phobias as snakes, heights, creepy-crawly insects or enclosed spaces were all significant threats to us as a species in our evolutionary past. Even water, before the popularity of swimming lessons and water sports, was a significant and common danger to us. In the same light, it is curious to note that the types and numbers of phobias are fairly constant and limited, consistently appearing among different populations around the world. It is also puzzling that we have few phobias of "modern" threats, such as guns and electricity. This fact has led to the theory that phobias are related to our evolution as a species, emphasizing that a proper respect for many of these dangers (heights, water, snakes) would be a protective response—individuals would "survive" better because they would have a stronger aversion or avoidance mechanism in reaction to these common dangerous stimuli.

In support of this theory, laboratory work has shown that children learn some fears more easily than others. For example, Rhesus monkeys raised in the wild are quite afraid of snakes—they undergo a marked anxiety change (increased heart rate, evasive behavior and agitation) in the snake's presence. However, monkeys bred in captivity (with no natural exposure to snakes) do not have this response. If the laboratory-raised monkey is exposed to snakes (or even pictures of snakes) while in the presence of a wild monkey (who has the typical anxiety or phobic reaction), the laboratory monkey quickly "learns" to react to the snake in an agitated manner. This reaction in the laboratory monkey is learned more quickly and lasts much longer than other conditioned responses, such as learning to avoid a flower or other innocent trigger that is associated with an electric shock. Somehow the laboratory-raised monkey is "prepared" or predisposed in some way to learn this specific phobia of snakes. The implication is that, for the monkeys, a healthy respect for snakes is an important evolutionary biological advantage that would protect the species. In Darwin's view the monkey who learns this "phobia" is fitter, more able to survive, and thus the trait is not only passed on, but also remains in reserve even in the brain of the monkey who has never been exposed to snakes.

In this way, it has been suggested that human phobias are evolutionary remnants, the result of a "prepared" conditioning of fear associated with objects and situations that have threatened us, especially our young. As a species, we might be more able, more "prepared," to learn or emphasize fear concerning such objects and situations. Those with phobias could simply be overreacting, biologically speaking, to important mechanisms in our evolutionary past that have allowed us to survive and be successful.

Blood/injection/injury phobia might also be an evolutionary remnant. In the animal world, when escape or defence is not possible, many prey species "freeze," becoming immobile, passive and inert. In spite of the imminent danger, their blood pressure and heart rate falls. Sometimes this results in less injury—the predator might give up the chase or exhibit decrease aggression when the prey is motionless. Physiologically, a drop in blood pressure and heart rate can mean less blood loss if injured; therefore, this pattern of freezing and fainting might allow a greater chance of survival.

Treatment
Specific Phobias
Most specific phobias can be effectively treated (without med-

icine) by exposure therapy, a program of gradual, progressively increasing contact with the feared situation or object. Often these sessions can be quite limited. For example, in one study 60 percent of individuals with spider phobia were treated successfully with a single treatment lasting two hours. The technique, called "flooding," consists of exposing an individual, under controlled circumstances, to the phobic stimulus in gradually increasing degrees until the anxiety starts to diminish. An important part of this technique insists that the individual control the exposure—not allowing the phobic stimulus to produce a full-blown anxiety attack, but only to produce mild symptoms that gradually abate as the object or situation remains. When the symptoms abate, the object or situation may be intensified or brought closer. For example, in the case of spider phobias, one protocol for treatment begins with an assessment of the cognition or "thinking" of the individual when anticipating seeing a spider. This important part of the protocol focuses on the anticipated fears (what the individual is afraid of), including such things as a bite from a spider, other injury, contamination, or just the feeling that the spider is "creepy-crawly" and moves unpredictably. Next, the individual is exposed to spiders—often beginning with such things as photographs, that the individual can look at and then handle. This usually produces some mild fear response (anxiety or tension) but with continued exposure, the anxiety usually begins to abate and the individual can carry on to the next step—a video or a movie of a moving spider (often it's the movement of the insect that is most distressing—it's unpredictable and rapid). Again, the movie or video is repeated until the anxiety is no longer overwhelming. Next, the individual is exposed to a specimen of a spider—perhaps a laboratory specimen of a large spider, such as a tarantula, preserved in a case. The individual is allowed to handle the dead spider in its protective box. Next, a live spider in a cage or case is introduced, and again the individual is allowed to observe the spider and eventually handle the case. Finally, the individual is encouraged to touch a live spider, or even, in some cases have the spider crawl over his or her skin.

Flooding works extremely well for most phobias, especially when paired with a cognitive behavioral approach to the problem. Controlling the physical sensations of anxiety is very important, and such relaxation techniques as yoga, progressive relaxation or breath control are very important to reduce anxiety symptoms during exposure. Because the combination of desensitization and relaxation is so successful, the use of medication is often not necessary in the treatment of phobia.

Blood/Injury/Injection Phobia

As we have seen, the physiologic response in this type of phobia is different, frequently causing fainting. Flooding can be used but, in addition, specific therapies are used to prevent the drop in blood pressure and heart rate that produce the loss of consciousness (see sidebar on page 75).

In a technique called progressive tension therapy individuals are taught to increase the tension in large muscle groups (such as the arms and legs) in order to maintain the blood pressure in a range that would prevent fainting. For example, individuals who are to have their blood drawn alternately flex and relax large muscle groups in the legs and arms before and during the blood taking. The contraction of muscle fibers increases the resistance to blood flow, prevents pooling of blood in the muscles, and increases the blood returning to the heart, thus raising the blood pressure and preventing the fainting episode. It is important to lie down when blood is being taken to prevent fainting; lying down helps prevent the drop in blood pressure as well.

SIX

Post Traumatic Stress Disorder

Even now, almost two years later, Joanne still could not recall all of the details of the accident, but she was certain of one thing—at least for a few minutes after the truck hit them, her mother had been alive.

It had been raining hard that November night, the explosive raindrops splattering loudly on the windshield. Joanne and her elderly mother had been grocery shopping and were heading home. As she approached a red stoplight at an intersection, Joanne reduced speed. She clearly remembers the light changing to green, and she proceeded through the intersection. Suddenly, a dark-colored pickup truck was right beside them, headlights blazing in through the passenger window. What happened next seemed to be in slow motion—in fact, Joanne had experienced it hundreds of times since that fateful night. She remembers trying to swerve, remembers the feeling of the blinding light filling up the car, of seeing her mother put her hands up in protection, and then the awful sickening feeling that they were about to be hit by the truck. This was the worst thing—the knowledge of the certainty of it, that they were no longer people—mother and loving daughter—but simply inanimate objects fixed in a very mechanical course of destruction. Joanne still can't recall the exact moment of impact, though she wasn't injured in the accident. She does remember her mother, sitting beside her in the car, head slumped down with blood dripping from her forehead. Fearing she was dead, Joanne screamed at her mother and shook her—she remembers quite clearly that her mother moaned in response.

The ambulance arrived shortly after an emergency crew pried open the passenger door, but it was too late. By that time, Joanne 's mother had died, her daughter helplessly holding her lifeless hand.

Since the accident Joanne had not been able to function— even though the doctor said she was not physically injured in the crash. She was unable to return to her work as a real estate agent, and, no matter how hard she tried, she couldn't function as a wife or mother to her two young daughters. She couldn't seem to focus, couldn't seem to get the accident out of her mind, couldn't concentrate, and couldn't seem to enjoy life. She frequently awoke at night sitting up in bed and crying— calling out her mother's name, reliving the crash.

And in any situation that was even remotely similar to the accident, she was paralyzed with fear and panic. For example, summer rainstorms filled her with dread and panic, as did any sudden bright light.

But the biggest difficulty was that Joanne was unable to drive the car. As a real estate agent, it was absolutely essential that she take clients out to properties and show them houses, but she was unable to travel in the car, even as a passenger. She was anxious sitting in the car even in the driveway, but as soon as the vehicle began to move, Joanne could not stand the feeling that she was about to have the accident all over again— she had to ask her husband to stop the car and she got out.

With her doctor's help, Joanne learned that she was suffer- ing from post traumatic stress disorder. The doctor was able to put a pattern to Joanne's behavior and explain that the event had been so emotionally traumatic for her that it had overwhelmed her sense of coping. With psychological therapy and antidepressant medication, Joanne was, over several months, able to return to work and to begin to reconstruct her life.

Since the beginning of recorded history, we have recognized that there are some events within the realm of human experience that are so disturbing, so threatening and so intense that those who experience them are forever changed. Each of us experiences hundreds of events and interactions every day, most of which are innocent, benign and consistent with the way that we understand the world to be. They are predictable, even expected events. Although not necessarily within our control, at least they "fit" into our conceptualization of how people should act, how we as individuals should react, and how the world, with all its natural laws and vagaries, should behave.

Unfortunately, some have experienced events that fall outside this norm, outside the way we understand the world and other people's behavior. Although we may be quite upset and disturbed soon after the event, most of us are able to incorporate it into a new understanding of the way the world works, and to process the event in light of this new understanding. We are able to move on, to remember the trauma as simply that—a memory of something bad that has happened to us.

However, for some of us, and for some particularly intense experiences, we are unable to move on, unable to process the event, unable to incorporate the event into a new understanding of our lives and the world. We are left with an intense feeling of unease and distress. Recurring fragmentary images of the trauma itself, with all the emotional reactions, intrude into our lives again and again, causing us to relive the difficult experience. Nightmares disturb our sleep. Days are filled with an increased sense of alertness or "jumpiness." All of these reactions leave us emotionally numb and fatigued, causing us to withdraw from enjoyment of life. This phenomenon is called post traumatic stress disorder (PTSD).

Diagnosis

PTSD is a psychiatric diagnosis, and several criteria must be met for the diagnosis to be made. These include:

- exposure to trauma, in which one experiences a feeling of intense fear or horror
- the trauma being repeatedly experienced in disturbing images, thoughts, nightmares, dreams or flashbacks
- psychological or physical distress on exposure to cues that resemble the trauma
- avoidance of stimuli associated with the trauma
- a general numbing of emotions
- symptoms of agitation and arousal, including insomnia, outbursts of anger, irritability and lack of concentration

The symptoms and signs listed above must be present for more than one month and must significantly interfere with the person's ability to function socially and occupationally.

Obviously, there must be a traumatic event, a distressing or emotionally disturbing experience (the word *trauma* comes from the Greek word *traumatos*, meaning wound). The event usually involves the threat of death, serious bodily injury or severe psychological damage. Of great importance is the feeling of helplessness, horror or intense fear that the trauma evokes.

An intense feeling of loss of control is another important feature. Although the trauma can be direct physical trauma

The terror of September 11

The destruction of the World Trade Center on September 11, 2001, was the largest single act of terrorism in American history. Almost 3,000 people were killed and the ten million New Yorkers living in Manhattan experienced the devastation firsthand. Surveys done soon after the event showed an increased incidence of symptoms of anxiety.

- One study done five to eight weeks after the attacks showed that the prevalence of PTSD in New York City was three times higher than usual.
- 37 percent of people who were inside the World Trade Center during the attacks had symptoms of PTSD.
- Almost one-third of the people in Manhattan who were diagnosed with PTSD did not directly experience the attack, but were reacting to television images and media coverage.
- Sixty percent of people living in Manhattan showed at least one of the symptoms of PTSD (the most common were intrusive memories and insomnia).
- In the months following the attack, there seemed to be a fairly rapid resolution of symptoms. One study done six months after the terrorist attack showed that PTSD had resolved in 50 percent of those showing symptoms.
- There was a heightened anxiety across the country. In one telephone study, done three to five days after the attack, 44 percent of Americans were bothered by at least one symptom of PTSD.
- Interestingly, there was no increase in prevalence of PTSD in Washington, D.C., where one of the hijacked planes crashed into the Pentagon.

(such as is seen in soldiers in wartime), it can also be indirect and emotional (such as the experience of watching a loved one die).

All who experience such traumas have difficulty handling them emotionally for some time afterward, but in PTSD the emotional experience, rather than being eventually relegated to our memory, is constantly re-experienced, with recurring images, sounds or smells suddenly appearing and intruding into our day-to-day lives. The experience is happening "all over again," the horror is relived. These so called "flashbacks" are recurring episodes that flood the mind with all the same emotional intensity of helplessness and terror that was felt in the original situation.

Flashbacks can be triggered by anything that even vaguely resembles the original experience. For example, a soldier hearing a car backfire on a quiet city street might suddenly feel that he is back in the battle zone, hearing gunfire, and feeling the imminent possibility of gruesome death. Flashbacks can occur when they are least expected and your guard is down— such as at first awakening, or after the use of alcohol. They are both disabling and distressing.

Most sufferers of PTSD try to stay away from any place or circumstance that might incur the intense emotional experience, and avoid conversations and experiences that might in any way resemble the original trauma. Such avoidance eventually produces a feeling of "numbing," a sense of detachment from others—that interferes with relationships and is a purely protective response. Sufferers often admit to a limited capacity for the enjoyment of life, friends and love. Many often have a pervasive sense of futility and assume that a shorter lifespan is their fate.

While the minds of PTSD sufferers might appear calm (because of their detachment), physical examination reveals that their nervous systems have been overstimulated. This phenomenon, called hypervigilance, reflects the fact that the trauma has produced a sense of increased alertness to the possibility of harm or danger, an increased watchfulness. It's as if the trauma has put the nervous system on "red alert," and the person is prepared to respond to the mildest stimulation; there is an overreaction to simple and common stimuli, such as loud sounds, bright lights, and even touch, with an exaggerated startle response, a "jumpiness" reflecting the fact that the body's response to sensory stimuli is markedly exaggerated.

Concentration is difficult (because sensory stimuli that would normally be easily filtered out, cannot be) and productivity suffers; falling and staying asleep is difficult. There are outbursts of anger or irritability, suddenly erupting without adequate explanation. The whole process is emotionally exhausting and reinforces the need of the person with PTSD to avoid any situation in which multiple stimuli might be present. Eventually, the individual becomes isolated, emotionally exhausted and chronically disabled.

What We Know About PTSD

The relationship between severe emotional trauma and disability has been known for centuries. In his epic poem, the *Iliad*, Homer described soldiers who returned from the Trojan War but were unable to function in their homeland because of psychological difficulty. Centuries later, survivors of the American Civil War were often seen to have the same psychological difficulties, with flashbacks and overwhelming anxiety, well described in Steven Crane's book, *The Red Badge of Courage*. The symptoms of palpitation, shortness of breath and acute anxiety were called "soldier's heart" by military doctors. The same phenomenon happened in civilian populations exposed to extreme trauma. In England, in the late 1800s, surgeon John Erichsen noted severe psychological problems resulting from injuries suffered on the railroad—such things as amputation or severe crush injuries—which he called "railroad spines," and that resulted in emotional disability, lack of concentration and inability to return to work. At the same time a similar type of psychological disability was described in females, often seen after severe emotional and physical trauma such as rape. This disability was called "hysteria," (the word comes from the Greek word *hyster* meaning uterus) and referred to the uncontrollable emotions (laughing, weeping and irritability) caused by grief or intense fear. Neurologist Jean-Martin Charcot described how severe emotional and physical trauma could put one in a mental state "similar to hypnosis," a state that we now call dissociation. He postulated that the state of dissociation—a feeling of not being physically present in a situation—is a protective phenomenon and the result of having endured unbearable experiences.

The global carnage of World War I provided many more cases of PTSD for study, as soldiers, prisoners of war, civilians living in combat zones, and others showed significant levels of psychological distress and disability. Terms such as *combat fatigue, war neurosis*, and *shell shock* were used to describe the nature of the emotional toll that war exacted. "Disorderly action of the heart" and "neurocirculatory asthenia" were medical terms coined to describe the intense anxiety and prominent cardiovascular symptoms. World War II produced many more cases of PTSD, but they were not always recognized as such. During this war, over 200 British soldiers were executed for "cowardice" (most, in retrospect, showing signs of the disorder).

Traumatic events that can lead to PTSD

- combat or war experience
- rape
- motor vehicle accidents
- death of a loved one
- physical injury (or threat of physical injury) such as assault, theft
- fire
- flood
- lightning
- earthquake or other natural disaster
- witnessing traumatic injury, suffering or death in others (especially loved ones)

The full understanding of PTSD had to wait for the Vietnam War of the late 1960s. In this war, not supported by much of the American population, many soldiers returned home but could not function because of flashbacks, the inability to concentrate, and other symptoms of PTSD. A group of psychiatrists in New York started holding rap sessions—discussion groups for returning veterans, so they could talk about their experiences. These initial discussion groups grew into an organized study of the psychological problems of veterans, eventually showing that 15 percent of Vietnam veterans suffered from PTSD, and a further 19 percent had many, but not all, of the symptoms.

In 1974, Ann Burgess, working at the Boston City Hospital, consistently observed similar symptoms in women who had been raped. She used the term *rape trauma syndrome* to describe the problem. As well, it was recognized that survivors of the horrific experiences in the concentration camps of Europe experienced the same flashbacks, numbing, emotional outbursts, and hypervigilance as the rape victims and the Vietnam veterans. Scholars began to understand that, although the traumas were different, the psychological reactions and disability were the same.

Over the years there has been a modification in the understanding of what type of event is sufficient to cause PTSD. Previously, psychiatrists felt that the event had to be "outside the range of usual human experience" and had to be "markedly distressing to almost anyone," but we now understand that the range of events that might produce PTSD is quite wide, including not only such things as rape, abuse, motor vehicle accidents, death of loved ones, fires, and floods, but also the witnessing of a traumatic experience (such as a car accident), occupational exposures (such as that experienced by police, firefighters and medical personnel) and a wide range of human experience.

Causes of Post Traumatic Stress Disorder

PTSD is a common psychiatric diagnosis, with a lifetime prevalence (the number of cases that are present in a population over a lifetime) of 7.8 percent. It is more common in women (about twice as common); men have a 4 to 5 percent lifetime prevalence and women have a 10 to 14 percent lifetime prevalence. It is the third most common anxiety disorder in the United States. Though at first glance it might seem that trauma sufficient to cause PTSD is unusual in our society, this is not the case. It has been estimated that at least 70 percent of American citizens experience trauma severe enough to produce PTSD. The usual causes include such things as the death of a loved one, interpersonal violence (rape, assault, torture), life-threatening events (such as motor vehicle collisions), and natural disasters (earthquakes, fires, floods), as well as combat. It is to be emphasized that, in the majority of cases, even severe emotional and physical trauma does not *usually* produce PTSD—most of us are able to survive the episode without long-lasting emotional consequences. However, there are several factors that make some of us more vulnerable to the development of PTSD.

The first factor is the nature of the trauma itself, with some experiences being much more likely to produce PTSD than others. For example, 55 percent of women who are raped develop symptoms of PTSD after two months. This figure drops to 7.5 percent of those who were in a motor vehicle collision and only 2 percent of those who learned of traumatic events (but were not actually themselves involved). The sudden, unexpected death of a loved one resulted in PTSD in 14 percent

Incidence of PTSD in various traumas

prisoners of war—67%
childhood victims of sexual assault—37.5%
adolescent survivors of serious motor vehicle collisions—34%
professional firefighters—18%
postpartum women—0.2%

of persons—the single most common traumatic event that triggers PTSD in both women and men.

One is more likely to develop PTSD if the stress:

- is prolonged
- is severe
- results in physical damage
- is grotesque or horrific,
- contains the threat of severe harm
- is unexpected (for example, police officers trained to respond to difficult situations have a lesser incidence of PTSD than civilians exposed to a violent crime)

In addition to these factors, a family history of PTSD (or any other anxiety disorder), previous severe trauma, lack of social support or disadvantaged socioeconomic status also seem to predispose individuals to the development of the disorder.

Co-Morbidity

Up to 80 percent of people suffering from PTSD have other psychological disorders. Almost 50 percent fulfill the criteria for major depression; dysthymia (a disorder related to depression), generalized anxiety disorder, panic disorder, and phobias are all commonly seen. In men, the most common co-morbidity is alcohol and drug abuse (seen in up to 50 percent), producing a dependency on these drugs as an attempt to treat the symptoms.

Women have a higher lifetime prevalence of PTSD than men though it is not clear whether this reflects an increased vulnerability to the disorder or the fact that, in our society, events are experienced differently. Women are more likely to be molested and sexually assaulted; however, men who are sexually assaulted have a higher likelihood of developing PTSD (65 percent versus 46 percent).

Understanding the Origins of Post Traumatic Stress Disorder

The Acute Stress Reaction

In order to understand why some of us develop PTSD, it is important to understand the process whereby we handle an acute stress or trauma. Much of the work on acute stress comes from wartime experience where the so-called "combat stress reaction" is a common problem. The emotional response of soldiers exposed to combat can include acute restlessness and anxiety, irritability, apathy, psychological withdrawal, increased startle reaction, abdominal pain, nausea and vomiting, and aggressive and hostile behaviors. Sometimes, paranoid reactions, distancy (thoughts of running away or returning to civilian life, or psychological numbing), and psychological withdrawal from the situation (dissociation) are seen. Loss of self-control, weeping, screaming, incontinence, disorientation and flight behavior are all common symptoms. For example, in the 1982 Lebanon war, combat stress reaction occurred in 25 percent of all Israeli casualties (similar statistics exist for the United States forces in World War II).

Studies show that if the trauma is severe enough (such as rape) symptoms such as these are, at first, almost universal but usually abate within time (remember, PTSD cannot be diagnosed unless the symptoms have been present for more than one month). Therefore, it is common and quite normal to experience flashbacks, increased irritability and nightmares in the immediate aftermath of such an event. However, in most people, these symptoms will eventually subside. In contrast, in PTSD people have a basic impairment in integrating the experience with other life events.

We now understand that severe trauma, or severe threat of trauma, has enduring biological, psychological and social effects, including a diminished capacity to deal with stress later in life. Exposure to severe trauma changes the brain in a predictable manner. Studies have shown that sufferers of PTSD have measurable and consistently observable changes in both the size of their brain structures and their functioning. It seems that, at the time of severe trauma, the excessive stimulation produces permanent neurological alterations within the brain. Somehow, the intensity of the experience combined with the severe emotional reaction that accompanies it are recognized immediately by the brain and handled differently from a more usual experience. It is as if the feelings of desperation and helplessness, of impending death or damage, are so marked that they "brand" the experience into the brain's circuitry, and that this "branding" actually damages the circuitry, altering the brain. In a home stereo system, if the volume of the music is turned up too loud, the speakers can be permanently damaged. A similar phenomenon occurs in those with PTSD. Studies have shown a decrease in the size of the hippocampus (the area of the brain responsible for short-term memory) and altered metabolism in the brain on PET (positron emission tomography) scans. The traumatic experience has been so vivid, so intense, that it has altered the brain anatomically and functionally.

In addition, the memories formed by such an experience are not "normal"—they are so intense that they produce only fragmented, but very vivid, "snapshots" of sensory experience, loaded with emotional context. The phenomenon is similar in the sense of "overload" to the home stereo speaker. In PTSD, the memories formed are qualitatively different—only parts of the memory remain (usually the most vivid), not a complete, organized, consecutive, flowing pattern. The memory cannot be shortened or expanded in detail or manipulated in other ways so that it can be described to others; it is often filled with "blank" areas, as though the person had not really been there.

Thus, the nature of memory formation in PTSD is completely different from the memory formation of a more benign event. In this latter situation, the memory can be incorporated into a regular understandable flow, including the progression of events as well as thoughts, images and feelings. The benign event memory can be adjusted—summarized or expanded in detail—for description to others. The memory can be understood clearly to be "in the past," completed and not recurring in the present. In contrast, the partial and abnormal memory formation in PTSD causes a permanent alteration of neurobiology that eventually produces the symptom complex.

Psychological Changes

Essentially, severe trauma in some people depletes the psychological resources needed to cope with life's subsequent experiences. By its very essence, the nature of trauma sufficient to cause PTSD is unpredictable, horrible and associated with marked or complete loss of control. The world is suddenly different—it has become a very unpredictable, unsafe place. The severe emotional response to the trauma leaves some of us emotionally depleted, and recovery involves redefining our world, accepting our fragility, examining the unpredictability of violence and evil, and questioning our understanding of the basic goodness of others (for example, after a rape). Our own evaluation of the traumatic event is critical in this process, as is the appraisal of those around us. Many such traumatic episodes involve a feeling of guilt, the feeling that we did not do "the right thing" or the honorable thing, that we were unable (for whatever reason) to change the situation or to rise to a higher ideal—such as sacrificing our own health or life for the safety of those around us. This so-called "survivor's guilt" seems critical, as the mind attempts to incorporate the experience into our own sense of personal value and meaning. Anger, sadness, humiliation and guilt are common. Many people blame themselves for some or all of the consequences of the trauma, and this sense of shame and loss of personal worth can be very prominent and very difficult to bear. The total loss of control over our destiny and the destiny and safety of others (particularly loved ones) leaves the person with PTSD in a state of perpetual psychological fear. This fear is so unpleasant that it quickly leads to avoidance behavior. Paradoxically, sometimes this leads to a desire to be exposed to the trauma again—in an attempt to "master" the situation that was so devastating. Thus, soldiers can become police officers or mercenaries. Commonly, the unbearable psychological symptoms come to the surface as physical complaints, such as headaches, abdominal pain, fatigue—a process known as somatization, and a common problem in medical offices, as those with PTSD often go to their doctors complaining of a collection of nonspecific but intense physical symptoms for which no medical cause can be found.

Biological Effects of Trauma

Exposure to acute trauma produces the full stress reaction in the body, including increased levels of catecholamines, corticotropin-releasing hormones and cortisol. Increased circulating levels of norepinephrine have been seen consistently in those who go on to develop PTSD. Norepinephrine, the "flight or fight" hormone, causes symptoms such as increased vigilance, increased alertness and "jumpiness," as well as physical signs such as increased heart rate, blood pressure, sweating and weight loss. People with PTSD may also have increased thyroid hormone levels.

In contrast to all other anxiety disorders, circulating levels of cortisol in PTSD are unexpectedly lower than normal. Levels of the corticotropin-releasing factor—the hormone that stimulates the adrenal gland to produce more cortisol—are increased. These measurements show that the person with PTSD biologically cannot contain the stress produced by the original trauma. The original trauma (the acute stress reaction) has caused such a depletion of the adrenal glands' ability to produce cortisol that they cannot "turn off" the stress reaction—and levels of catecholamines and norepinephrine remain quite high. Thus, there are predictable, measurable and consistent biological changes (both within the brain and within the hormonal system) that explain the symptoms and signs of PTSD.

Opioids Produced by the Body: Endorphins

Intense fear or trauma can cause the secretion of endogenous (meaning with no external source) painkilling compounds produced within the brain; these opioids help to produce some blunting of the emotional response, as well as pain relief (called stress-induced analgesia). When secreted, these protective chemicals allow us to survive events, such as personal physical injury, by blocking the pain that we might feel. It is as if, in certain extreme situations that are simply too much for the brain to take, your body has a mechanism to ease the pain. These chemicals are responsible for heroic acts of valor and physical activity (such as being able to walk on a broken leg) during times of excessive stress. It is believed that they are at least in part responsible for the phenomenon of dissociation.

Dissociation is a response to acute stress that produces a disconnection, a separation (in the mind) from the extreme situation. Dissociation can be seen in panic disorder, but is commonly seen in acute severe stress, and is more common in children. Survivors describe a feeling that they are watching events from a distance, outside the body, looking at themselves and their problems much more objectively, with a feeling that what is taking place is not really happening to them but to someone else. Similarly, survivors describe "blanks" in their memory—times that they were not aware of what was happening, although to others they seem to be functioning. These blanks are thought to be a psychological mechanism for handling severe trauma or injury. Sometimes this dissociative state persists after the trauma and often interferes with everyday functioning.

Prevention of PTSD

As we have seen, PTSD is, in many situations, predictable in its incidence, depending to a large degree on the nature of the trauma and the vulnerability of the person traumatized. Primary prevention efforts (such as gun control, enforcement of traffic laws, the prevention of child abuse and sexual and domestic violence) play a large role in decreasing the chance of exposure to a particular trauma. In addition, studies have been done to see if psychological counseling or "debriefing" might help those exposed to severe trauma by decreasing the incidence of PTSD.

While at first these studies did show some benefit, with survivors having fewer symptoms a short time after the trauma, recent studies have suggested that psychological debriefing might in fact increase the incidence of PTSD. In two recent studies— one on patients in burn units and the other on patients involved in motor vehicle accidents—those people who had debriefing had a higher incidence of PTSD.

Currently, it is felt that those people who experience a stressful event and develop symptoms soon after, and who thus have a greater chance of progressing to PTSD, should be treated with more intense counseling. Studies have shown that those with acute stress reaction showed more than a 50 percent reduction in the incidence of PTSD when they were so treated. Psychological debriefing might, therefore, be useful in order to determine who is at higher risk for developing PTSD.

Treatment

Although complex in its biology and psychology, PTSD is quite treatable, with various studies showing success rates up to 80 percent. Usually, pharmacological agents (such as SSRIs, SNRIs or the tricyclic antidepressant clomipramine) are combined with cognitive behavioral therapy (focusing on insight and exposure to cues of the previous experience). Attention to lifestyle issues (such as alcohol use) and anxiety management reduction techniques (such as exercise, yoga or other relaxation techniques) are an important part of the treatment. An unusual form of treatment is eye movement desensitization and reprocessing (see sidebar on next page.)

Eye movement desensitization and reprocessing

One of the most interesting developments in the behavioral treatment of anxiety disorders is the Eye Movement Desensitization and Reprocessing technique (EMDR), in which the patient imagines a frightening or disturbing image while carefully following the therapist's finger as it moves back and forth across the visual field. EMDR grew out of the experience of inventor Dr. F. Shapiro. While remembering some of her own traumatic memories, she realized that her eyes spontaneously shifted from side to side. She noted that this combination caused a marked decrease in her emotional distress. The technique has been used with PTSD as well as panic disorder. It is now felt that other sensory stimulations (such as listening to tones or other sounds played in alternate ears) may have the same beneficial effect. There is no universal agreement as to the mechanism by which the method works, but, in some patients, it can produce fairly dramatic results, without any significant side effects.

SEVEN

Obsessive-Compulsive Disorder

As soon as he awoke, Keith knew that today was not going to be easy: it was the day of his performance review at the factory. Keith wasn't worried about the review itself—he'd worked at his canning machine for years—but he was quite concerned about all the people he would be meeting for the review, including the personnel director, his supervisor and the owner of the factory. That meant shaking their hands, and Keith didn't like that. Even now, on awakening, he was worried. He was frightened that, overnight, while sleeping, he might have touched somewhere on his body that would have contaminated his hands. He wore underwear and pyjamas to bed just to be sure, but he couldn't know exactly what his hands had touched overnight. The more he thought about it, the more he was certain that his hands were filthy, and this made him feel uncomfortable and distressed, even though he knew his fears were unreasonable. On the way to the bathroom, Keith kept his hands upright, the way a surgeon does when preparing for the operating room, opening the door with his foot. He didn't want his hands touching the door handle, leaving microscopic germs that might contaminate him the next time he had to use the door.

In the bathroom, Keith had a specific routine for cleaning his hands. First, he slowly filled the sink with water that had to be just the right temperature—not too hot, but warm enough to kill bacteria. Next, Keith took a small amount of liquid soap, carefully measured in the palm of his left hand and began, very precisely and slowly, to wash the fingers of his right hand beginning with the thumb. Keith knew that the thumb was the most important finger, and also the filthiest one, and thus it had to be cleaned very vigorously and with attention to detail. Keith's hands were dry and sore from repeated washings but he persisted, assiduously and slowly washing the thumb inch by inch, beginning at the nail (where he imagined germs and grime might remain hidden and protected).

Standing by the sink, washing his thumbnail, Keith thought about the upcoming meeting, with all the people involved. He usually tried to avoid meeting people, and especially touching them by shaking hands. He felt very agitated by the possibility that one of the others might have hands contaminated by filth, or sweat, or worst of all, excrement. He couldn't imagine that they would be as careful with cleaning as he was. It would be impossible to clean his hands right away—after all, the handshaking would take place at the beginning of the meeting— and Keith, standing in front of his bathroom sink, shuddered to think of the diseases that they may be carrying—diseases like hepatitis or meningitis or even HIV. Just the thought of it filled his mind with dread. He could imagine himself dying in a hospital bed, his flesh wasted, his body rotten and smelling. Keith knew that his chances of being infected were slim, that he was exaggerating the risk; nevertheless, the thought filled him with disgust. He felt so uncomfortable that he scrubbed harder and harder until his thumb began to bleed.

Obsessions—Anxiety-Producing Thoughts

Obsessive-compulsive disorder (OCD) is the combination of obsessions (anxiety-producing thoughts), and the actions (compulsions) taken in an attempt to reduce this anxiety.

An obsession is an unwanted and upsetting thought that intrudes into the mind repeatedly. An obsession could be an idea (such as Keith's fear of contamination or infection), a feeling (for example, that you have to straighten the silverware on the dining room table), a picture or image (for example, an image of cars colliding), or an impulse (for example, the thought that you might want to shout out obscenities during a prayer in church). Obsessions are unpleasant and very disturbing; they create a feeling of extreme anxiety, unease or distress. They recur frequently, often in the same form or shape, and each time, they persist for some period—they are not simply fleeting thoughts that are quickly gone from your mind. They demand your attention and prevent you from focusing on anything else; even though you recognize that the obsession is unreasonable or exaggerated, you cannot dismiss it. You are certain that the thoughts arise from within your own mind. Although obsessions often come from a trigger, they are usually not related in a realistic way to the worries of everyday life.

Obsessions are different in quality and intensity from normal worries and concerns. From time to time we all have disturbing thoughts or images that enter our mind—usually caused by situations of stress and real life problems. Such worries are usually reasonable concerns based on some degree of truth or experience and, although they produce some distress, they are usually fairly easily dealt with by using logic and reason. For example, it's not uncommon for parents to worry that their child could be harmed in traffic on the way to school. A very disturbing image of an accident scene, with the injured child, might fleetingly appear—but most parents are able to place the thought in its proper improbable context by reasoning that the child will walk on the sidewalk and cross the street with a crossing guard. Consequently, while the thought is emotionally disturbing, it can be thought through and resolved.

Obsessions are far more powerful and demanding, and cannot be banished simply by using logical analysis, nor can they be ignored or suppressed. Obsessions usually produce a much more emotional response. They are often repugnant, disgusting or extremely frightening, producing severe feelings of anxiety, dismay or dread. Although obsessions can arise from everyday stresses (such as Keith's meeting with his superiors) they are usually an unreasonable exaggeration of risk or reality, and are recognized as such.

The appearance of an obsessive thought is often preceded by a trigger—either external, such as an object that one sees in the environment (for example, Keith might see a stain that triggers his fear of contamination), or an internal thought or experience (for example, Keith's anticipation of the meeting). An obsession is passive, it comes without being asked; it is a thinking process that produces anxiety. The only way to reduce and respond to the extremely uncomfortable distress produced by an obsession is to engage in an action or activity, called a compulsion.

Compulsions—Anxiety-Reducing Actions

A compulsion is an action or behavior performed in response to an obsession. Compulsions are usually purposeful, voluntary and repetitive activities performed either to reduce anxiety or to prevent some dreadful event or consequence—they are the actions taken in response to the extreme distress produced by an obsessive thought. Compulsions are not reasonably connected to the observed thought or obsession (for example, a person might have to find a specific series of numbers in the morning newspaper in order to prevent an accident on the way to work). They are often clearly inappropriate or excessive to the situation (for example, Keith washes his thumb until it bleeds in order to prevent infection). Compulsions are not passive, but active: one chooses to perform them. They are often complicated and intricate, with many steps and procedures that must be executed in a very specific and precise manner, as in a ritual, and they make the person with OCD feel better. The specific sequence, details and exactness of the compulsion is an important part of its effect on reducing stress. If the act is interrupted, or not performed in its specific rigid manner, the compulsion does not reduce stress and, therefore, must be repeated in order to have the desired effect.

Thus, a cycle develops. A trigger (either internal or external) prompts an obsessive thought that produces intense, unbearable anxiety and distress that, in turn, is reduced by completing a compulsive act.

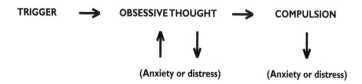

Both obsessions and compulsions, although they can have a superficial basis in truth or life experience, often have a magical or unbelievable aspect that gives the individual unrealistic power. Two examples are a mother feeling that harm might come to her child if certain numbers are not found in the newspaper each and every morning; or imagining the violent death of a loved one if a convoluted ritual, such as cleaning all the household knives in a certain order, is not completed. Compulsions, although they are often physical movements or activities, can also be confined to mental tasks, such as counting backward or repeating religious phrases or sayings. Sometimes compulsions take the form of an excessive need for symmetry or order, hoarding of worthless objects, or even excessive slowness in the performance of everyday tasks, such as dressing, washing or showering.

Diagnosis

The psychiatric diagnosis of obsessive-compulsive disorder is defined as being the presence of obsessions and compulsions that occur frequently (they take up more than one hour a day), and are severe enough to interfere with an individual's normal routine, employment, and/or social functioning and relationships. Also, the patient must realize that the obsessions or compulsions are not realistic—that they are unreasonable or not connected in a realistic way to life experiences or real life problems.

It is important to differentiate between the psychiatric definition of obsession and compulsion and common usage of these words. Often the word *obsessive* is used casually to describe a mental fixation on a specific idea or problem ("he's obsessed with the idea of failing"). This can be normal behavior—the idea of failing becomes an important fear—but it doesn't interfere with the function in other aspects of life. Similarly, meticulous or perfectionist tendencies toward orderliness, fastidiousness and precision are perfectly normal (and indeed laudable) traits that are often very helpful in everyday life. Obsessive-compulsive disorder is different in quality and intensity from normal fastidiousness, and rather than helping a person to be successful, it interferes with normal functioning.

Who Gets OCD?

Obsessive-compulsive disorder is common, with a lifetime prevalence of 2.5 to 3 percent (about one person in forty-five). Between four to six million people in the United States are affected. It is twice as common as schizophrenia. In adults, it affects males and females equally—although in children, males predominate (they seem to have an earlier onset of the disorder). Although it can be seen in children as young as age two, it most commonly appears in the late teens or early twenties, with a mean onset of 19.8 years. Two-thirds of cases appear before age twenty-five and it is unusual for the disorder to begin after age thirty-five. The onset is often fairly sudden, and 50 to 70 percent of individuals describe some sort of stressful event (such as the birth of a child, the death of a family member, financial or personal strain) associated with onset. However, in up to 40 percent, no such specific event is recalled. Hormonal change in women (such as a pregnancy) can precipitate or exacerbate the disorder. Obsessive-compulsive disorder is usually a lifetime problem. In only 8 percent of individuals do the symptoms abate without treatment. Although the disorder can be intermittent, 80 percent of those with OCD have continuous symptoms and disability.

How Does Obsessive-Compulsive Disorder Affect Life?

Some individuals with OCD can have fairly normal lives, but many find the quality of their lives severely altered. Recurring obsessions produce overwhelming anxiety and a state of chronic emotional distress and exhaustion. Fear, chronic worry and anxiety become daily ordeals. Anger and irritability are common results. Overwhelming disgust, paralytic fear and chronic stress are very disruptive to emotional health. Consequently, relationships with family and loved ones suffer. In

Does perfectionism produce OCD?

Perfectionism, the characteristic of aiming for faultlessness and excellence, can be a valuable personality trait, motivating a person to great achievement by demanding a high standard of performance and accountability. Perfectionists often have extraordinary expectations of themselves and others, intolerance for errors or mistakes, and a strict sense of order and precision about their world. They can be very difficult to live with. However, as demanding and difficult as this personality trait might be, it is not obsessive-compulsive disorder. Perfectionism often confers a social advantage in that the perfectionist might achieve more because of the trait. Social functioning and interpersonal relationships are not disrupted by the tendency—in fact, life might very well be better because of the accomplishments. This contrasts with OCD where the pattern of behavior interferes with both relationships and functioning. In addition, there is no evidence that those individuals with perfectionist traits are more liable to develop OCD than the general population; perfectionism is different from OCD and does not produce it.

addition, compulsive acts are often complicated and time-consuming activities, sometimes bizarre in quality, and can lead to physical injury or illness. The cycle of obsession and compulsion spoils life, leaving the sufferer emotionally and physically unable to participate in social relationships or employment opportunities.

In one study, 43 percent of individuals with OCD never married. Severe restriction in contact with others is common. Poor academic or school attendance and performance can limit career choices as can specific compulsions; for example, an obsession with contamination would prevent a teaching career because children might need physical contact, such as the washing or care of an injury.

Secrecy, shame and withdrawal are common, as the individual realizes that his or her behavior is not appropriate or understandable to others. The distress of obsession is so acute that the avoidance of situations that might trigger obsessive thoughts is paramount; therefore, social events, such as family encounters or trips to the shopping mall, are minimized or avoided. The experience of life is truncated.

Family members and/or friends are often drawn into the process, which can complicate the situation because their own needs and feeling are affected. They are often asked to adapt to the obsessions, and to help by participating in the compulsions, sometimes with bizarre or unrealistic actions. The sufferer might not be able to prepare food, wash clothes, or take out the garbage, and friends and family, trying to help, find themselves doing more and more in an intricate pattern of support.

Marjorie's family wondered if their mother was getting Alzheimer's disease. At seventy-six years of age, she was still living in the family home, but since her husband's death, her behavior had become more and more bizarre. Marjorie's greatest joy in life had always been her family, and she loved being involved in their birthdays, graduations and special events. Now, however, it was very difficult for her family to get her to leave her home at all, and when she did, she wasn't happy. They all realized that the responsibility of looking after the house loomed large in Marjorie's mind, but they couldn't understand why she felt so uneasy when she was away from the home. Constantly, she wondered aloud whether the house was "safe," whether she had left on one of the burners on the stove or whether there was anything else that might go wrong during her absence.

Last weekend, when the family gathered to celebrate Marjorie's granddaughter's ninth birthday, instead of participating in the child's celebration, Marjorie insisted that she had to be taken back to her home. She was very upset, fearing for certain that she had forgotten to lock the front door, leaving the home empty, and available to any "robber or criminal." When it was pointed out to her that she had already checked the door (with her daughter who picked her up for the birthday party), Marjorie still could not be settled, could not believe that the house was secure. Eventually, to calm her, they left the party early.

At the family doctor's office Marjorie's memory testing was normal—she didn't have Alzheimer's disease. The diagnosis of obsessive-compulsive disorder was made and treatment initiated with psychological counseling and antidepressant medicine. Marjorie was soon able to begin to enjoy her family once again.

Co-Morbidity
As in the other anxiety disorders, co-morbidity with other psychiatric problems is very common. Major depression is seen in 50 to 65 percent of individuals with OCD, and social phobia is seen in 25 percent. Alcohol and substance abuse is very common—the drugs are used as a way of reducing the anxiety produced by obsessions—and often complicates the course of the disorder. Specific phobias, panic disorder and eating disorders are also seen.

Common Patterns of Obsessions and Compulsions
Theoretically at least, the list of possible obsessions and compulsions should be endless, with as much variation as there are personalities within the world, but this is not the case. Remarkably, across cultures and countries, only a relatively small number of combinations are commonly seen. Individuals can have multiple obsessions (and compulsions) but there is usually a common fear or concern—a theme, as it were—to their disorder (such as that of cleanliness). Though it is most common

Superstitions versus OCD

If you spill salt at the dining room table, do you throw a small amount over your left shoulder? If you make a comment about your good fortune, will you knock on wood to prevent something bad happening? Would you feel uneasy if you couldn't find any wood?

These are examples of superstitions—irrational beliefs based on fear of the supernatural, the unknown or the mysterious. Often based on religious or historic beliefs, superstitions are a very common part of our culture and have at their root a desire to affect the course of the future by some specific activity. Although sometimes they can predict a positive change (finding a penny will bring good luck), most superstitions are associated with preventing some negative outcome (avoiding the cracks on the sidewalk will ward off bad luck). Psychologists tell us that superstitions are more prevalent in those who overestimate the threat of negative events, yet who do not feel fully in control of their circumstances; superstitions increase during times of stress, such as war or natural disasters. Engaging in the superstition can create the feeling of bringing some control to your life. The superstition always implies a cause-and-effect relationship between what you do and the dire circumstance you are trying to avoid; for example, if you do boast of your good fortune and do not knock on wood, this will "cause" the good fortune to end. To a much lesser degree the distress of not finding wood to knock on mimics an obsessive's anxiety. Those with global anxiety disorder often report that worrying about a feared event made it less likely to occur—that is, the worry itself prevented the event.

A major distinction between superstitious individuals and those with significant anxiety disorder is that of disability. Superstitions might temporarily disrupt your day, but anxiety disorders, by definition, interfere with social and occupational functioning, often as a consequence of their

to have obsessive thoughts followed by compulsive actions, some individuals have obsessions without compulsions. This phenomenon is called rumination, the excessive inappropriate obsessive thought not followed by any sort of behavioral or mental act or compulsion and thus little relief of the anxiety. Compulsions without obsessions are rarely seen but can occur with greater frequency in young children (for example, repetitive hand washing). Let's look at some common patterns.

Contamination

The fear of contamination, "of being dirty," infected, impure or diseased is one of the most common obsessions in adults and certainly the most common obsession in childhood (in one study 85 percent of children with OCD and 60 percent of adults with OCD had this complaint). Contamination concerns can be focused on a wide variety of objects, substances and illness including:

- germs
- bacteria
- excrement or other human waste (such as sweat)
- chemical radiation
- environmental pollution
- household items
- animals or insects (cockroaches or flies)
- sticky substances or residues
- illnesses such as cancer or HIV/AIDS

These obsessions produce a strong and irrational fear that disease will result from contact with any of these substances, unless adequate cleaning takes place. Compulsive washing of hands, the most common obsessive reaction, is frequently excessive (sometimes more than 100 times a day), methodical and aggressive. Sometimes, people go to dermatologists or emergency room physicians with injuries to their hands from the repeated scrubbing and cleaning. Extremely time-consuming, repetitive, complicated, and excessive cleansing routines are common, and include:

- precise showering, bathing
- dry cleaning

- removal of waste
- personal grooming or toilet routines
- cleaning of households (counters and floors)
- cars
- clothing
- pets

Cleaning materials, such as cleansers or detergents, are used to excess, as are tissues, toothpaste, soap and even toilet paper. Specific areas of the house (such as the washroom), utensils (such as the broom or mop), even certain anatomical regions (such as the feet or the genitals) are meticulously avoided, as are situations or places where contamination might occur. Irrational beliefs about the consequences of contamination are common. Sigmund Freud described how one of his patients would iron his paper money "to destroy the germs" and thus prevent infection. Individuals have a concept that bacteria and disease lurk everywhere, simply waiting for a chance to infect, and this drives the need for excessive cleanliness.

Intrusive Thoughts

In this, the second most common pattern, obsessions take the form of thoughts or images of harm to the self or others. These images are often horrific, with violent, frightening or disgusting images or feelings. For example, an individual might see himself running over a pedestrian while driving, feel certain that this has happened, and, consequently, might drive the same route again and again, looking for signs (such as an ambulance or police) to confirm his suspicion. The image can be particularly gruesome and horrible. A mother fears she has harmed her newborn baby by suffocation or stabbing, producing unbearable distress. Sometimes the obsession is of a sexual nature with thoughts or images of sexual encounters with a variety of people not usually expected (for example, children, in-laws, the elderly). This pattern of obsessions leads to compulsions, such as penitent acts of prayer, counting, mental checking or organizing, or repeated motor activities, such as walking or driving the same route, again and again.

Checking and Pathological Doubt

In this type, insecurity is the trigger for obsessions of doubt and concern, often focused on everyday events or circumstances. For example, constantly doubting that the door has been locked, the stove or kettle turned off, or food returned to the refrigerator produces a daily feeling of anxiety and fear. The doubt can be quite bizarre—for example, not being sure that you hadn't stabbed someone overnight in your sleep. The doubt is not reasonable, and cannot be easily relieved except by compulsive checking of doors, locks, utensils or electrical appliances, and even then the obsession is not dispelled. This leads to bizarre repetitive behaviors; for example, despite constantly going back to the house (not trusting your judgment or observation) you are still left with an uncomfortable feeling of guilt and negligence because specific tasks might have been forgotten, thus risking catastrophic consequences that could cause damage or illness to others.

Symmetry—Slowness

In this variant, there is an overwhelming need for symmetry, precision and order, and marked distress if this is not achieved. This is a fairly common pattern in children, who are very upset when, for example, the dinner table is not set "just so" with everything in its exact and proper spot. This leads to compulsive acts of ordering and arranging objects that can be quite bizarre (for example, a child refuses to travel in the car unless everyone else in the family sits in their "usual seats"). Primary obsessional slowness is a variant of this need for symmetry, in which simple everyday tasks (often self-care tasks) are performed in a ritualized and precise manner, taking up an inappropriate amount of time. It seems as if the task (such as cleaning one's teeth) is not the important element, but rather the performance—the task must be completed exactly and correctly—is the important goal. Even while realizing that it is not reasonable to spend such an amount of time on the task, such people perform sequential, complicated time-consuming routines without question. The obsession is actually the need to be extremely meticulous and the compulsion is the activity or behavior that results. For example, the routine task of brushing your teeth is broken down into its component parts (exactly the right amount of toothpaste on the toothbrush, exactly the right amount of water) and component actions (focusing on one tooth at a time), often to a ridiculous degree, such that showering or bathing, shaving and dressing can take up to four or five hours out of the day.

Other Types

Compulsive hoarding, in which individuals show an inability to discard worn out or worthless objects even when they have no sentimental value, is a compulsion more frequently seen in the elderly. In this variant, obsessions of not being adequately prepared for the future are sometimes seen, but the compulsion of excessive acquisition is the usual manifestation. Sometimes hoarding can be bizarre—for example, searching out garbage for treasures, buying excessive household supplies "to be sure I don't run out" or compulsive buying (for example, of newspapers). Sometimes the objects saved may be quite unusual — such as hair caught in the hairbrush or fingernail clippings, but often the objects are those used in everyday life—newspapers, plastic bags or pieces of cloth. The collecting is clearly excessive and often dangerous enough to constitute a health risk with such things as huge piles of newspapers or other objects interfering with cleaning the home or proper hygiene. While hoarding can begin in early life, it becomes more of a problem in the elderly. In one study, 40 percent of complaints to a public health unit about hoarding involved the elderly. Interestingly, hoarding seems to be seen more frequently in those who were, in some way, deprived in their early years; it is more common in Holocaust survivors and abused children.

Religious obsessions are also seen and frequently focused on blasphemy (such as shouting out swear words during prayer) or in contrast, excessive morality. Religious obsessions are more common in those with a religious upbringing, and the particulars of the obsession and compulsion vary with the religious practice.

Trichotillomania, the compulsive pulling out of hair, associated with tension or an irresistible urge before pulling and followed by pleasure or relief, is another common compulsion. It can result in significant hair loss and disfigurement. Individuals often cannot identify a specific intrusive thought (obsession) but simply say they feel an increasing sense of tension or stress that is relieved by the activity. The hair pulling is not felt to be painful, but rather pleasurable. Any hair-bearing area on the body may be affected, including the eyebrows, eyelashes, armpits, and pubic hair, as well as scalp hair.

Body dysmorphic disorder

In this disorder, preoccupation with a minimal defect in physical appearance produces significant distress that interferes with the quality of life. Individuals focus on perceived or minor abnormalities of their body (particularly on the face) with unrealistic assessment of the impact of these minor defects. For example, the nose may be too "inflated," the chin may be "not well developed" or the eyes may be "too close together." The concern is not that of normal, reasonable examination of one's features, but rather an intense unrealistic evaluation of a minor defect. Individuals perceive that others are judging them by the defect, staring at them and repulsed by them. Thus social and interpersonal relationships are often affected. Attempts at masking or hiding the perceived defect (such as makeup or plastic surgery) are common. The disorder is amenable to treatment with both psychotherapy and pharmacological agents.

Causes of Obsessive-Compulsive Disorder

When this disorder was first described in the seventeenth century, the person's symptoms were felt to be the result of possession by an evil spirit or force, and the treatment was exorcism. We now understand that the disorder is the result of a combination of factors, including genetics, brain chemistry function and anatomy, and environmental triggers—both mental and physical.

There is no doubt that, as in other anxiety disorders, there is a genetic tendency or predisposition to the problem. Relatives of individuals who suffer from OCD are five times more likely than the general population to have a similar problem. In the studies of identical twins (who have exactly the same genetics), if one of the twins develops OCD, the chance that the other twin will develop it is ten times greater than in the normal population—implying a huge genetic predisposition.

Biochemists have shown that in OCD there are abnormalities in the neurotransmitter serotonin, one of the chemical messengers involved in transmitting information from cell to cell within the brain. In addition, the brains of those suffering from OCD are anatomically different—small groups of cells in the brain stem called the basil ganglia (and especially the caudate nucleus) are smaller than usual, as shown on magnetic resonance imaging. Other studies show an increased activity in the frontal lobes (the site of insight and planning). Why these changes occur is not known. There could be some psychological experiences that predispose to the development of OCD. It has been theorized that an early sense of responsibility in children, strict enforcement of disciplinary codes or religious zeal, or a family environment that overly emphasizes the possibility or threat of danger in the world might foster the development of OCD in those already genetically predisposed.

Physical environmental factors might also play a part. Some studies have shown an association between streptococcal infections, the common "strep throat," and the development of OCD in children, suggesting that, in some susceptible individuals, the body's immune response to the streptococcus infection might alter brain function to produce the disorder. This is not as fantastic as it sounds; there is another neurological disorder that is well understood to be a consequence of streptococcal infection in some children. Doctors noted years ago that some children with a streptococcal throat infection developed involuntary dance-like movements of the arms and legs, a condition called chorea. The movements would become gradually more severe, affecting all motor activities including walking, lifting and grasping objects, and speech. The complication, now known as Sydenham's chorea (after the physician who first described it) is known to be a transient brain dysfunction produced by the body's response to the streptococcal infection. In a process known as "molecular mimicry" the antibodies that the child produces to the streptococcal infection interfere with function of the anatomical regions of the brain responsible for movement. In addition to the dance-like activity, some children also develop psychiatric symptoms. The same type of mechanism might play a part in the development of OCD. Some children have had a fairly dramatic onset of obsessive-compulsive symptoms shortly after a streptococcal infection; one-third of these children have movements of Sydenham's chorea, suggesting that the same phenomenon of antibody "mimicry" could be producing the onset of OCD. Because streptococcal infection is so common and this information is only fairly recently available, it is difficult to estimate what percentage of OCD could have been produced by this infectious mechanism.

Treatment

As a general statement, OCD is quite responsive to treatment. Long-term studies show improvement in over 90 percent of people treated with a combination of pharmacological and psychological therapies.

Pharmacological

Because dysregulation of the serotonin neurotransmitter system is felt to be a significant part of the biochemical mechanism for symptoms in this disorder, the use of chemicals that aid in the control and regulation of this system has been associated with marked improvement. SSRIs, SNRIs and some tricyclic antidepressants (particularly clomipramine) that act on the serotonin system have been particularly useful and are the usual pharmacological treatments. Lithium and the MAO inhibitors (especially phenelzine) may also be used.

Cognitive Behavioral Therapy

CBT is considered to be an essential part of therapy. This may take the form of individual or group sessions focusing on understanding the problem, challenging false or escalating beliefs, desensitization, reassessment of inappropriate responses and the institution of control. Family involvement is often very beneficial.

Other Treatments

Electroconvulsive therapy may be used for extreme cases that do not respond to other treatments. Surgical treatment (a procedure known as stereotactic psycho surgery) may be used in cases resistant to all other treatment. In one study surgery was successful in treating 26 percent of people who otherwise did not respond to treatment.

EIGHT

Anxiety in Children and Adolescents

There was no doubt about it—William was not going to school again today. Although he'd been in school for several years, getting him to attend had always been a struggle. Often, before school, when he complained of stomach pain or a sore throat, his mother had realized that he needed comfort and reassurance. She was usually able to get him to go to school and, once there, the teacher generally reported that the rest of the day was fine. But not today. William had complained of a stomachache soon after awakening, and, when his mother tried to get him to go to school, William began to cry, and then shout and scream, flailing about with amazing force. They were now a full week into the school term, and William had not attended once.

He had always been what his mother referred to as "an emotional child," needing more reassurance and support than her other children. For as long as she could remember, he had had difficulty sleeping, had imagined ghosts and demons in the room, and had been able to sleep alone only during the last year. This past week his sleep had been even more disrupted—

often he was unable to get to sleep until well past midnight. Last night, he'd gone into his parents' room saying that he just simply "could not sleep."

While his mother was unwilling to physically lift him up, put him in the car and drive to school, she was nonetheless distressed that he was missing school. She had no idea why he was so upset or what she should do.

Normal Anxiety of Childhood

Fear and anxiety are both normal in childhood. In many senses, part of growing up relates to the development of appropriate respect for the dangers of this world and an appreciation of how fragile life can be. Such understanding is part of what compels children to take responsibility for their actions, to anticipate consequences and to value relationships. In short, fear and anxiety help youngsters to mature and develop into adults.

Newborns know neither fear nor anxiety, but toddlers are universally upset when their primary caregivers leave. Young children fear the dark, imagining danger in their bedroom, and, around the world, school-age children have concerns about their performance at school and their social relationships. Usually, children master these fears with the passage of time, and, with the development of self-esteem and independence, are able to cope with the fear, put it in its proper place and perspective, and continue their development. This process of adaptation is age specific; that is, the usual fears of a two-year-old are mastered by the time the child is seven.

Unfortunately, children are not immune to anxiety disorders—conditions in which the anxiety is not manageable. These fears differ from normal childhood experiences in two ways: they are much more intense and protracted than normal, and they disable the child by preventing normal activities and functions. All of the anxiety disorders are seen in childhood, and many of them typically begin in childhood and adolescence. Because of children's youth and lack of experience, and because their ability to vocalize thoughts and feelings are not fully developed, the way they talk about or exhibit these disorders is significantly different from adults.

When Children Have Anxiety Disorders

As in adults, when children have anxiety disorders, they have a combination of physical and psychological symptoms as well as changes in behavior. Bodily complaints are very common and include:

- headaches
- abdominal pain (for which no medical cause is found)
- insomnia
- recurring sore throats
- fatigue or "not feeling well"

Psychological symptoms include:

- "what if" questions—"what if you get hit by a car ...?"
- frequent worrying about bad things happening, a constant fear or concern, inability to be reassured
- intrusive thoughts "I've got to wash my hands" (obsessions)
- unreasonable fears of insects, animals, heights (phobias)

Usually anxiety disorders in children cause observable changes in behavior such as:

- clinging, not willing to let a parent out of their sight.

Does your child have an anxiety disorder?

A Parent's Checklist
- Are there recurring symptoms of headache, abdominal pain, dizziness or shortness of breath?
- Is there insomnia?
- Is there repeated, persisting questioning about "bad things"?
- Is there repeated avoidance of activities that are appropriate for the age of the child?
- Is the child excessively timid or easily frightened?
- Is there ritualistic behavior—the insistence on specific detailed sequences of actions and subsequent distress if these are not followed?

- avoiding situations that produce anxiety (for example, refusing to go to school)
- tantrums or "freezing" in a difficult or feared situation
- insisting on doing things "just so" in a ritualized manner, and being very upset if unable to
- ritualistic (specific, repetitive behavior) activity
- episodes of sudden severe disabling fear (panic)

Causes of Childhood Anxiety
The current understanding is that anxiety disorders are the result of both a genetic predisposition and life experiences. Thus, a child may be "programmed" with a tendency toward anxiety problems, and the child's ability to cope with this tendency can be compromised by an external stress in her or his life. For example, it is not uncommon to see stressful events, such as moving to a new neighborhood or changing to a new school, as the trigger for an anxiety problem. Similarly, peer interactions, bullying, poor performance at school or excessive pressure for high achievement can precipitate difficulties. The more significant the event (for example, divorce or death of one parent), the higher the chance that the child will have some

anxiety difficulties. Understanding these stress factors, and dealing with them, is an important part of treatment.

Specific Anxiety Disorders in Children
Separation Anxiety

This is defined as an abnormal, disabling anxiety in a child who has excessive fear relating to separation from a parent or loved one, or from home. It is the most common anxiety disorder in childhood and, although it can occur in younger children, it reaches a peak incidence in seven to eight-year-olds. Three to 4 percent of all primary school-age children and 1 percent of adolescents have the problem.

Some anxiety about separation from loved ones is, of course, quite normal. At about nine months of age, infants begin to show signs of distress when separated from their primary care-giver. Similarly, some anxiety is normal when children first leave home to go to school or camp, or sleepovers with friends. However, separation anxiety is diagnosed when *excessive* anxiety develops at an age when it is not usually seen, and is accompanied by symptoms of unwarranted worry, nightmares, repeated physical complaints, and refusal to go to school (or to be separated). The anxiety caused by these situations can be very severe, approaching panic. Also, temper tantrums and bizarre behavior, such as hiding, throwing things or rage attacks, can be seen. It appears to be more common in children who are easily embarrassed or timid.

To be diagnosed with an anxiety disorder, symptoms must be present for more than one month and must interfere with the child's functioning. Treatment usually involves psychological counseling, and is usually quite effective.

Selective Mutism

This anxiety problem is diagnosed when the child will not speak in a certain social situation in which speaking is expected, even though speech is normal in other situations. Commonly, the child speaks normally within the nuclear family, but refuses to speak at school or in some other social situation. Sometimes the child will communicate with non-verbal gestures (such as shrugging or pointing). Obviously, this interferes with the child's performance and function. Some degree of mutism is extremely common in children who attend school for the first time. Sometimes, children might whisper instead of speaking properly. Selective mutism is not uncommon, occurring in 3 to 8 children per 100,000, and is more common in girls and those with delayed speech onset. In most cases, it is felt to be a symptom of social anxiety disorder (one study found more than 90 percent of children with selective mutism had social anxiety).

The diagnosis of selective mutism can be made only after the child has had symptoms for more than a month that are not limited to the first month of school. Treatment, focusing on social skills and the development of self-esteem, is usually very effective.

Trichotillomania

This term refers to the recurrent pulling out of hair, producing noticeable hair loss. Usually, an intense sense of tension or anxiety precedes this activity, and it is the action of pulling the hair that produces a feeling of relief, pleasure, gratification or calm. Although scalp hair is most often pulled, any hair on the body (including pubic) can be involved. Sometimes the pulled hair is put in the mouth and swallowed.

Stuttering

Defined as a disturbance the flow and timing of speech, stuttering is a common problem, in both children and adults. The repetition of sounds, the interruption of speech or the insertion of pauses that disrupt the flow of speech are the common patterns. It is seen in 1 percent of the adult population and commonly begins in childhood—often between age two and three years. Interestingly, it does not begin suddenly; its onset is gradual. It is four times more common in males than in females.

The relationship between anxiety and stuttering is complex. While there is no evidence that anxiety or stress causes stuttering—stutterers have no more psychiatric difficulties than others—it is well known that, in those who have the problem, stuttering is much more frequent and disruptive in situations of stress. In addition, stutterers fear the stuttering itself, often avoiding situations or even words where stuttering is more likely to be triggered. Stuttering is usually treated with a combination of speech therapy and relaxation techniques.

The syndrome usually begins in childhood or adolescence, and is often associated with other anxiety problems, especially OCD. Treatment is aimed at addressing the underlying anxiety disorder.

Panic Episodes

While most panic episodes begin during or after puberty, they are not uncommon in younger children. Depending on the age of the child, physical symptoms (such as sudden shortness of breath or dizziness) can predominate, leading to the diagnosis of asthma or some other breathing difficulty. Children do not often complain of the abnormal thought patterns of panic (such as the fear of dying or of losing control), but rather the physical symptoms predominate. Avoidance behaviors are very common (for example, not wanting to go to school for fear of an attack). Nocturnal panic attacks can be hard to distinguish from nightmares. Panic episodes in children are usually treated with cognitive behavioral therapy.

Specific Phobias

Phobias are very common in children, especially animal and blood or injection phobias. In one study, the average age of onset was four years. Situational phobias (such as the fear of heights) begin later, usually in late adolescence or early adulthood. A child with a phobia might exhibit "freezing" behavior, obvious irrational fear, temper tantrums, screaming episodes, excessive clinging or nonspecific avoidance behavior (for example, refusing to go to camp). Some phobias might be learned (or at least encouraged) by observing a parent's response to a certain situation. For example, seeing a parent react hysterically to the presence of a cockroach, the child might "learn" this as an appropriate response.

Treatment in children involves the same measured and gradual exposure to the phobic agent as used in adults. Success rates are high.

Social Anxiety (Phobia)

Although the peak age of onset of this disorder is in the teen years, it is not uncommon to have a diagnosis in a child as young as age five. Unlike adults, children often do not realize that their anxiety or fear of being scrutinized by others is excessive or irrational. They simply respond to a situation by being easily embarrassed, shy and generally unable to function. Crying episodes, temper tantrums, withdrawal from social situations and avoidance (such as refusing to go to school) are quite common, often limiting the child's social encounters, school performance and the development of self-esteem. Selective mutism is more common in social anxiety disorder. Treatment, aimed at understanding, from a child's perspective, the difficulties and gradually teaching the child coping mechanisms is often very effective.

Generalized Anxiety Disorder

The exact age at which this disorder starts is often difficult to pinpoint. However, those with it often report that they were "anxious" or "worriers" all their lives. The syndrome is frequently first noted by others in adolescence, as the excessive anxiety and worry interfere with the young person's performance. In young children insomnia, clinginess, and excessive apprehension and worry about everyday events (as well as catastrophes) are the usual presenting symptoms. Physical symptoms (such as headaches or abdominal pains) are often prominent, leading to multiple visits to the doctor and investigations.

Treatment, aimed at understanding the disorder and focusing on cognitive behavioral therapy, is often very successful.

Obsessive-Compulsive Disorder

The mean age of onset of this disorder is twenty years; however, it can be seen in children as young as two. In children with this problem, boys outnumber girls two to one while in adults the numbers are equal. Commonly, affected children do not realize that the obsession-compulsion complex is unreasonable or excessive. Being unable to verbalize their emotions, they often have difficulty explaining why they have to behave in a specific manner. Frequently, the problem comes to light because of ritualized behaviors—specific rigid activities that must be performed in a certain way and that often take an inordinate amount of time. Sometimes the problem shows up because family members are unwilling to participate in the rituals (for example, parents insisting that the child go to bed without arranging all the toys in the room in a specific manner). Because an obsession that is not followed by a compulsion produces a very uncomfortable feeling, crying, temper tantrums, shouting matches and even rage attacks are not uncommon. These children seem to be "angrier" than other children, more irritable and easily upset. Treatment with a combination of cognitive behavioral therapy and sometimes medicine is usually very effective.

Diagnosing and Treating Anxiety Problems in Children
If you think your child might have an anxiety disorder, see a doctor. Making the diagnosis on your own is very difficult. Anxiety problems can be caused by certain medicines (decongestants or inhaled salbutamol for asthma), drugs (caffeine in soda pop, chocolate and cocoa), or by other medical disorders (such as hyperthyroidism). Physical symptoms (such as abdominal pain and headaches) need appropriate medical investigation.

A doctor's first step in deciding the appropriate treatment is the attempt to understand the child's situation, particularly the level of stress that the child perceives. Many anxiety disorders begin after a specific external stress (such as the death of a grandparent or moving to a new neighborhood). In these situations it is important to pay attention to the specific stressor. Grief counseling, speaking to the teacher, preventing bullying behavior and evaluating the child's total stress load could all be appropriate first steps before prescribing medicines.

Psychological Therapy
Anxiety disorders in children respond to psychological therapy, just as those in adults do. Obviously, the approach and technique must be modified for the child's age, level of development and understanding. Cognitive behavioral therapy (CBT), adapted to the specific child, is very effective in treating many

of these difficulties without the use of any medications. CBT addresses the physiological symptoms, the cognitive changes and the behavior seen in the disorders, and targets each of these to produce change. For example, a child with anxiety commonly believes that something "bad" will happen at school but, by exploring this belief, the child can be reassured. Relaxation techniques can be extremely effective even in very young children, as can desensitization techniques.

Medications

In some severe anxiety disorders in children or in those not responding to psychological therapy, medications can be considered. SSRIs are usually the first-line medications. As always, the benefits from the medications must outweigh their risks—but some anxiety disorders are so severe, and so disruptive to a child's normal functioning and maturation, that the medicines can be helpful. It is important to target specific symptoms in the treatment, to be certain that these improve, and to establish an individual dosing pattern.

Two possible side effects of SSRIs are worth noting. Agitation is seen in some children when the drugs are first introduced, requiring the dose to be reduced. In addition, there is some concern that the risk of suicide may be increased in young people on these medicines. Health Canada has issued a warning to physicians, suggesting that the medicine has an increased risk profile for this problem.

Benzodiazepines, although they may be used for short-term relief of symptoms (such as the prevention of a panic attack in a specific circumstance) are not usually used longterm in children.

It is important to emphasize that the diagnosis and treatment of anxiety disorders in children and adolescents allow the young person to mature and grow without the added stress of these problems. Anxiety disorders, once recognized, can be effectively treated.

NINE

Treatment for Anxiety Disorders

Anxiety disorders are chronic problems—left untreated, most will not simply go away but will persist over a lifetime. Through daily distress, they result in years of suffering and pain. Many individuals with these disorders suffer in ignorance, unaware of the medical nature of the syndrome that is so negatively affecting their lives. Others suffer in silence, afraid to reach out for help because they fear the stigma of being labeled "mentally ill." Still others are unable to access trained personnel to help.

Treatment of any anxiety problem begins with knowledge; understanding the nature and particulars of the disorder, how it behaves and how it affects you is the first step in getting better. Just realizing that there is a pattern to the symptoms you suffer, and that you are not alone, can lift a weight off your shoulders.

This chapter is about treatment. Specifically, it is about the particulars of treatment (such as psychological therapy and medicines) that you can use to supplement your own learning and self-help methods. Explore the resources available at the end of the book (see page 164). Join self-help groups for people with similar problems. Attend lectures and information sessions about anxiety. Many people feel that self-help workbooks are a very effective way of learning about anxiety problems and beginning to change your approach to them.

See your doctor. Your family doctor can confirm your diagnosis, interpret your problem in the light of any other medical problem you may have and begin to treat you. Often psychologists or psychiatrists may be used as consultants to help in your treatment.

It needs to be stressed that anxiety disorders are *very* treatable, allowing you to regain control of your life, and ultimately, your happiness.

Treatment often does not rely solely on one approach. Frequently, it can incorporate psychological therapy, behavioral therapy and sometimes medication. Let us explore these various treatment options.

Cognitive Behavioral Therapy

This treatment program, now well accepted as being effective for anxiety disorders, is based on the concept that our feelings and our actions are a direct result of the way we think or react in a particular situation. For example, if we spend much of our time worrying about dreadful possibilities of harm or danger to our families, then we will feel anxious and fearful most of the time and we will behave in a tense and frightened manner. This is not a new idea. Two thousand years ago, the Greek philosopher Epictetus wrote, "it is not things themselves that disturb men, but their judgments about these things," emphasizing that it is not an event in itself that determines how we react or behave in a situation, but rather our "thoughts" or assessment of the event. In addition, the way we feel (and the way we behave) affects the way we think. For example, if we feel sad or depressed most of the time, we begin to think that things are hopeless. Thus, these three elements—thoughts, feelings and behavior—are interlinked, each able to affect the other.

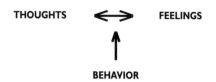

Cognitive behavioral therapy uses this understanding to challenge and then change the thinking and thus both the feelings and behavior.

Cognitive Therapy
Shakespeare wrote "there is nothing either good or bad, but thinking makes it so." Cognitive therapy is based on the premise that changing the way we think about a situation or event (our cognition) will change the way we feel (our emotions or mood) and ultimately our behavior. The way we think about a situation is often a result of our previous experiences ("every time I go to the movies I have a panic attack") and our beliefs or assumptions ("the world is a very dangerous place—accidents can happen at any time"). Cognitive therapy usually begins by teaching the nature of the anxiety disorder—the pattern and the particulars, then focuses on an individual's thinking and assessments. Some examples of distorted and unreasonable thinking (or cognition) patterns are:

- all or nothing thinking—seeing things in black or white terms; if it's not perfect, it's awful

- unhealthy or negative self-talk—"I can't do this ... I'm a failure ..."
- overgeneralizations—seeing a single negative event as confirmation of defeat in life
- catastrophization—each disappointment, no matter how minor, is seen as a catastrophe
- mind reading—automatically assuming that someone thinks badly of you (with little justification for this thought).
- fortune telling—"knowing" that things will turn out badly, and then behaving accordingly
- accentuating the negative—ignoring positive events and exaggerating negative ones
- self-blame—using guilt to motivate yourself; unfairly blaming yourself for something bad that has happened

Through this process, an individual becomes aware of the pattern of negative thinking. By challenging and reconstructing this awareness, individuals can decrease anxiety. All of the anxiety disorders will respond to this type of treatment, although it is particularly helpful in social anxiety, panic disorder and general anxiety disorder.

Behavioral Therapy
Behavioral change goes hand in hand with cognitive change—individuals learn to behave (to act) differently in situations of stress, developing new ways of dealing with issues and events. This therapy usually begins with an assessment of how the individual reacts (or behaves) in a particular situation, in order to identify a pattern of behavior—and then progresses to adjust this pattern of behavior. For example, in social anxiety disorder, where individuals fear scrutiny from others, specific situations (such as meeting new people) are identified, and

specific techniques (such as learning to shake hands, repeat and remember names, and make small talk) are learned and then practiced, in order to help decrease anxiety and stress. Obviously, the behavioral changes will be specific to the anxiety disorder and to the individual, but learning new reactions in situations helps reduce the feeling of stress.

Behavioral therapy is particularly effective in panic disorder and social anxiety disorder.

The Effects of Cognitive Behavioral Therapy (CBT)

When she arrived for her first session with the psychologist, Susan was skeptical. She had difficulty believing that it would be possible to stop her panic attacks "just by talking." However, she realized she needed to do something to stop these dreadful episodes, or at least to minimize their effect on her.

The psychologist began by asking Susan about herself—her background, her family, her job. Then, together, they focused on the history of Susan's panic attacks, particularly their onset. They had come at a time when Susan was under a great deal of stress. Her mother had just recently been diagnosed with breast cancer, and Susan had recently received a promotion at work. After reflection, Susan began to understand that this was, in fact, a period of high stress for her, and that this elevated stress level was a significant daily force at the time her panic attacks began.

Next, Susan and her psychologist began to discuss the attacks. Susan was able to describe them in great detail: they always started with a strange feeling of unease, then quickly progressed to shortness of breath, then palpitations. Soon afterward Susan would feel completely incapacitated—sweating and trembling, unable to focus or concentrate, even becoming so dizzy that she would fall to the ground.

With the psychologist's help, Susan began to realize that there was a common pattern of presentation to her episodes: they always began with the feeling of unease, the shortness of breath, etc. She discussed with the psychologist the places that the panic attacks frequently occurred (crowded rooms, during exercise). Susan learned more about panic attacks by reading information provided by her psychologist. She learned that her attacks were "classic;" that she was not alone. She learned that what seemed like a meaningless pattern of progression was quite common. This understanding was quite a comfort to Susan, who up until this point believed that she was suffering a unique and personal problem.

In subsequent sessions, Susan learned to careful dissect the various symptoms of her panic attack. She learned to separate the feeling of shortness of breath from the palpitations, the dizziness and the other symptoms. She recognized that, in the past, she had not been able to stop the progression from one symptom to the next. With the psychologist's help, she learned that her rapid breathing might be contributing to the problem; that hyperventilation can change the chemistry of the body, producing sweating and trembling. She learned that, at the beginning of a stressful time, if she began to hyperventilate, she could produce a full-blown panic attack.

With her psychologist's help, Susan tried to experience some shortness of breath without progressing to a panic attack. She practiced being short of breath (by doing things like running up stairs) right in the office. At first, she was very frightened, afraid that the familiar symptoms would lead to a full-blown attack. She was relieved and pleased with herself when they did not. The psychologist led her through a technique of relaxation and muscular relaxation. Susan felt quite calm as she learned these steps.

Over several sessions, Susan learned about panic disorder, began to understand why it would happen to her, and, more importantly, learned to prevent her panic symptoms from progressing to a full-blown attack.

CBT has proven to be a very effective way of treating anxiety disorders, either when used by itself or, as is frequently done, in combination with medication. When used alone, it can be very effective treatment for some anxiety disorders (for example, up to 75 percent of individuals with panic disorder can be effectively treated with CBT alone), and some elements of the therapy are used as standard practice for all of these disorders. Unfortunately, intensive CBT (that is, therapy on an individual basis over an extended period of time) is not readily available and can be expensive. The treatment is usually provided by a psychologist or psychiatrist, and often extends over a period of many weeks.

Herbal Treatments

Interest in herbal medicines has grown dramatically over the last few years, as individuals seek safer and more natural products to deal with anxiety and other medical problems. One American study showed that 42 percent of those surveyed used some form of complementary or alternative therapy—and 31 percent of those used these treatments for anxiety. The following herbs have been used to treat anxiety disorders.

- **Chamomile:** The flower heads of this plant, used since Roman times as a tea because of its calming and digestive effects, do show evidence of a mild effect in reducing anxiety, helping with sleep, and decreasing inflammation in the skin and mucous membranes. It is very safe, with few side effects reported, but it usually has only a mild effect.

- **Kava:** This herb, a derivative of the pepper plant, is mixed with coconut milk and used as a traditional social greeting of welcome on many South Pacific islands. Served in a half coconut shell, the gray liquid has a calming, mildly sedative effect. In clinical trials, there is evidence of benefit for anxiety disorders. In spite of this evidence, kava should not be used, because the drug has been associated with changes in liver function and, in some cases, liver failure (hepatitis, cirrhosis and liver failure necessitating fulminant liver transplant). Accordingly, Health Canada has advised that products containing kava should not be used. This is not a problem of efficacy but rather of safety.

- **Passion flower:** The aerial parts of this plant have been shown to be helpful in mood disorders with anxiety, although there are few clinical studies. It also has mild sedative properties. There have been reports of an altered sense of reality in a few patients taking the herb. Drowsiness can occur.

- **St. John's Wort:** This herb, derived from the golden flower of the plant, has been used for the treatment of depression and anxiety as well as for the healing of wounds and burns for more than 2,000 years. There is evidence for its usefulness in depression and anxiety disorders; it is thought to act like an SSRI. It can also help insomnia and restless sleep. Unfortunately, it can interfere with the action of many common medicines including warfarin (decreasing its effectiveness), digoxin (decreasing the level of digoxin in the blood) and oral contraceptives, among others. It can cause an increase in liver enzymes and mild gastrointestinal symptoms. It should not be taken with antidepressants. It can produce photosensitization, the appearance of a rash in skin exposed to sun, a phenomenon first noted in fair-skinned cows that grazed in fields where St. John's wort grew freely.

- **Valerian:** The root and rhizome of this garden heliotrope has been used for years as a mild, safe sedative. It can be used for treating insomnia and for the relief of anxiety. It has been used in managing withdrawal from benzodiazepines. It is usually well tolerated with minimal side effects causing less of a hangover than benzodiazepines and no effect on alertness.

A Warning

Herbal medicines, though derived from natural sources, are often complicated chemicals with multiple effects and interactions. Most are not approved for use in pregnancy (objective data of their safety in pregnancy is lacking). Many herbal preparations interfere with other medicines (see, for example, St. John's wort); please tell your doctor if you are using these.

Medications

Although many anxiety disorders (especially phobias) are best treated with counseling, education and behavioral therapy, your doctor might choose to use medications to help treat your anxiety symptoms. The action of many of these drugs is within the brain, at the site where individual nerve cells communicate one with another.

The brain weighs only 1.5 kilograms (3 pounds), but it contains over 100 billion nerve cells, and each of these cells is in contact with many other cells, allowing communication and coordination. It is at the site of contact (called the synapse) where most of the medications used for anxiety exert their affects. Brain cells don't exactly "touch" each other physically in the synapse—they are separated by a micro space, a space that is filled with a liquid "soup" of chemicals. When an electrical impulse or message comes from one nerve cell, the impulse must cross over this soup-containing space to transmit the impulse to the next nerve cell. This transmission of information from one cell to another in the synapse is facilitated by chemicals called neurotransmitters (literally chemicals that transmit information from one neuron [nerve cell] to

Nerve Cell Communication

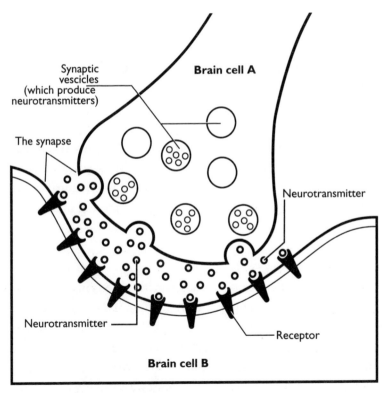

The space where two brain cells touch—the synapse—is the site of action for many anxiety medications.

another). There are many different types of neurotransmitters within the brain, but the neurotransmitters serotonin, norepinephrine, gaba and dopamine are critical in anxiety disorders. The concentration of neurotransmitters between the two cells is crucial in allowing the cells to communicate, to "talk to one another." The neurotransmitters are produced by the first cell (the cell with the "message"), then released into the soup to carry the information to the second cell. The neurotransmitters are then taken back up into the first cell (reabsorbed) or chemically degraded in the soup. Anxiety disorders are associated with dysregulation of these neurotransmitter systems, and many medicines helpful in these disorders affect the concentration or duration of action of these chemicals.

The following medicines are commonly used in treating anxiety disorders.

Antidepressants
It might seem odd to use antidepressants in anxiety states, but the syndrome of clinical depression is also associated with altered levels of neurotransmitters, and these chemicals have proven to be very effective in reducing and managing anxiety, as well as depression.

Tricyclic Antidepressants
This group of chemicals—named for the three rings or cycles in their molecular structure—was originally prescribed for depression, but is now frequently used for anxiety disorders (generalized anxiety disorder, panic disorder, post traumatic stress disorder, obsessive-compulsive disorder), as well as eating disorders and chronic pain. They work by reducing the uptake of the neurotransmitters norepinephrine, seretonin and others.

There are many different drugs within this class, and several (especially clomipramine, desipramine, imipramine and amitriptyline) are effective in anxiety disorders. They are usually quickly absorbed, have a half-life of about one day in the bloodstream, and can be very helpful in the treatment of anxiety disorders.

Side effects include sedation, dizziness, tremors, fatigue, weight gain, sweating, gastrointestinal symptoms (especially constipation), blurred vision and sometimes fainting. They should be used with caution by people who have heart disease and glaucoma. They can be used as first-line treatment in post traumatic stress disorder (amitriptyline or imipramine) and obsessive-compulsive disorder (clomipramine).

Selective Serotonin Reuptake Inhibitors (SSRIs)
Fluoxetine (Prozac), introduced in 1988, was the first of this new class of antidepressants. Since then, the drugs have been used by more than 12 million people worldwide. Although originally prescribed for depression, drugs in this class are now indicated for treatment of all the anxiety disorders (except specific phobias). They work by increasing the amount of the neurotransmitter serotonin available in the chemical soup between brain cells. They do this by blocking the uptake of serotonin back into the original transmitting cell—hence their name, selective serotonin reuptake inhibitor.

They are effective and usually well tolerated but may have side effects including nausea, anorexia, agitation, dizziness, abnormal dreams, irritability, headache and diarrhea. Sexual dysfunction is not uncommon. This group of drugs can produce decreased libido in both sexes as well as an inability to achieve orgasm in females, and impotence and delay (or failure) of ejaculation in males.

Specific Types of SSRIs

Fluoxetine: This drug has a half-life of two to three days, but its active metabolite has a half-life of seven to nine days. This means that the drug takes a long time to clear from the body (it may take one to two months for complete clearance). Because it is metabolized by a specific chemical pathway (cytochrome P450) it may interfere with other medications. It can produce agitation, headache, insomnia, sweating, dizziness and weight loss.

Citalopram: The half-life of this SSRI is about thirty-seven hours. Although it may cause nausea, dry mouth, headache, diarrhea, somnolence and sweating, it's less likely to interfere with other medications.

Fluvoxamine: This SSRI, with a half-life of fifteen hours, has more of a tendency to produce sedation, often of benefit in an agitated patient. Sleepiness can be a side effect. It should not be taken with decongestants (such as terfenadine or astemyzole).

Paroxetine: The half-life of this SSRI is about twenty-four hours. Weight gain, sleepiness, nausea, constipation and sweating are the more common side effects. Interactions with other medicines can be a problem.

Sertraline: The half-life of this SSRI is twenty-six hours. It also tends to be more sedating than some of the other SSRIs. Sleep disturbance, tremor, sweating, diarrhea, nausea and drowsiness can been seen as side effects.

The SSRIs are often effective in treating anxiety, but stopping them quickly is commonly associated with symptoms of dizziness, vertigo, lethargy, muscle pain, tremors and insomnia. In addition, a rapid increase in anxiety with agitation and crying might be seen, as well as reduced concentration. Even a short period without the drugs—for example, a weekend—can produce these symptoms as well as sudden electric-like "shocks" when turning the head quickly, flashing lights and vivid dreams. Accordingly, these drugs should not be discontinued suddenly, but rather the dose should be carefully and progressively lowered under direction from your physician.

Buspirone
This drug, the only drug in its class, is used for the treatment of anxiety disorders, especially generalized anxiety disorder. It acts on the serotonin receptors in the synapse, producing a calming effect. In contrast to the benzodiazepines, it does not have any sedative or muscle relaxant effect. It has a low potential for abuse, does not impair cognition and does not increase the effects of alcohol; it is rapidly absorbed, with a half-life of two to eleven hours, necessitating taking a dosage two to three times a day, and takes about four to six weeks to achieve its full effect.

There might be side effects of headache, nausea, dizziness and insomnia. It is effective for generalized anxiety disorder but can be used in post traumatic stress disorder as well. It does not seem to be as effective for people who have previously been treated with benzodiazepines.

Venlafaxine
This relatively new drug works in the synapse between nerve cells by inhibiting the uptake not only of serotonin, but also of norepinephrine and (to a lesser extent) dopamine. It is rapidly absorbed, with a half-life of only five hours, but is

available in an extended release tablet. Originally designed for depression, it is also effective in all of the anxiety disorders, but most commonly used in generalized anxiety disorder. The most common side effects include nausea, somnolence and insomnia, although dry mouth, dizziness, nervousness, constipation, and abnormal ejaculation or orgasm might be seen. A significant side effect is increased blood pressure, seen with greater frequency as the dosage of Venlafaxine increases. For example, in one study, 13 percent of those receiving more than 300 mg of Venlafaxine a day had significant hypertension. Thus, pre-existing hypertension is a relative contraindication, and all patients should be checked for this problem while using the medicine.

Monoamine Oxidase Inhibitors
These drugs are also used as antidepressants. They work by inhibiting the breakdown of neurotransmitters in the synapse by interfering with the action of the enzyme that chemically changes these transmitters—an enzyme called monoamine oxidase. These drugs are not used as frequently now as they once were because of the risk of their side effects—particularly an increase in the neurotransmitter norepinephrine when foods containing the precursor of norepinephrine (a chemical called tyramine) are eaten. In this situation, there is no enzyme to break down the excess norepinephrine produced from the ingested tyramine, and over-excitation, elevated blood pressure, headache and rapid heart rate result. Because tyramine is found in many foods (cheeses, beer, smoked meats, soya sauce, avocados), strict dietary restriction is necessary when on these medicines.

A drug called moclobemide is a newer drug in this class; it produces a reversible block of the monoamine oxidase enzyme and, although it can cause a dry mouth, blurred vision and headaches, strict dietary avoidance of tyramine-containing foods is not necessary.

Benzodiazepines

These drugs are among the most commonly prescribed drugs in the world. They work in the synapse at a binding site for the neurotransmitter GABA (gamma-aminobutyric acid). As a class, these drugs have properties to decrease anxiety, to sedate (to calm, quieten), to decrease excitability, to produce muscle relaxation and to facilitate sleep by producing drowsiness. In anxiety disorders these drugs are often used to reduce the daytime distress of anxiety, and also to help with sleep.

There are many types of benzodiazepines; some of the more common ones used in anxiety disorders are listed in the table. Because they are rapid acting, their calming effects are beneficial particularly at the initiation of treatment.

Common Benzodiaepines

Drug	Usual Dosage	Absorption Rate	Half-Life
Alprazolam	.25–.5 mg	medium	12 hr (short)
Clonazepam	.5–2 mg	rapid	36 hr (long)
Diazepam	5–10 mg	rapid	100 hr (long)
Lorazepam	1 mg (does have sublingual)	medium	15 hr (short)
Oxazepam	15–30 mg	slow	8 hr (short)

Side effects of benzodiazepines include oversedation, drowsiness, dizziness, unsteady gait and decreased vigilance. All of these symptoms are made more potent by the use of other chemicals that can produce sedation (for example, alcohol or over-the-counter drugs, such as antihistaminesor cold tablets).

The use of benzodiazepines for a short course of treatment (one to two weeks) may be very effective in anxiety disorders, but longer-term use is often complicated by the presence of tolerance and withdrawal symptoms. Tolerance refers to the phenomenon that the same dosage of drug no longer has the desired effect—the calming or "relaxing" effect of the benzodiazepine is lost with the passage of time as your body adapts to the medication—so you need to progressively increase the dose of the drug to produce the same effect. The body has become "tolerant," or used to the original dose so the effect is lessened. In addition, discontinuing the dose of a benzodiazepine (particularly if the drug has been used for some time and your body has become used to functioning with the medicine) can produce withdrawal symptoms—your body is "different" without the drugs, producing symptoms such as increased anxiety, headache, insomnia, shaking and sweating. Benzodiazepines do not treat depression, a problem commonly seen in association with anxiety disorders; in some individuals they can produce or exacerbate depressive symptoms. For these reasons, benzodiazepines are not usually recommended as first-line treatment for anxiety disorders, but rather as an adjunct treatment particularly in the beginning of treatment.

Although medications can be effective in all of the anxiety disorders, they are particularly useful in the treatment of obsessive-compulsive disorder and post traumatic stress disorder. They are often used in conjunction with cognitive behavioral therapy and supportive counseling. Medications are usually prescribed by medical doctors (either family physicians or psychiatrists).

TEN

Taking Back a Sense of Control

ost people who suffer from an anxiety disorder find themselves overwhelmed by a complex, seemingly random pattern of extremely distressing feelings and symptoms over which they have no control. These problems occur frequently without warning and produce marked disability. As a result, people with these disorders feel confused and angry, at the mercy of these intense, emotional events. In addition, they often feel it's their "fault"—as if there was something in their makeup that either caused the problem to appear or, more frustratingly, that if they only tried harder they could somehow control the symptoms. They are left with a sense of feeling assaulted by the disorder: they didn't deserve it, yet are powerless to prevent or control it. Loss of self-confidence—even loss of self-worth—is a common reaction.

This chapter is designed to allow you to begin to take back some control of your life. Tremendous advances have recently been made in the understanding and management of these common disorders, allowing individuals to master the problem and begin to enjoy life once again.

The First Seven Things to Do

Learn All You Can

1. The first step in beginning to conquer an anxiety disorder is to learn all that you can about the condition. You have already begun that process by reading this book. The knowledge empowers you—it gives you a pattern, an organization to the events and symptoms that seemed before to be random. The more that you learn about the problem, the greater will be your sense of control. Knowing that you are not alone, that you did not deserve to have the problem (but, in most cases, were simply genetically predisposed), will enable you to distance yourself from the disorder, protecting your sense of self-value. You are not a "panic disorder" or any other diagnosis. Use the resources at the end of the book to obtain further information and support. Make a point of attending seminars and self-help groups, and using workbooks, which have been shown to improve anxiety disorders. Knowledge is power.

Exercise

2. There is excellent evidence that exercise, by itself, will help reduce anxiety disorders. This calming effect is seen at any age and with both aerobic and anaerobic exercise (although aerobic exercise seems to have a more beneficial effect). Good exercise should produce a peaceful, calming effect on your body—after all, you are simply letting your body do what it was designed to do. Simple, noncompetitive exercise, done at an intensity that is comfortable, is a pleasurable, almost relaxing phenomenon. Ideally, exercise should be something that you enjoy, not something that you "have to do." Activities such as walking, slow jogging, bicycle riding

or cross-country skiing are ideal. Simple games of tennis or lawn bowling are also helpful. Highly competitive or intense activities (such as squash or hockey) are not relaxing for many people with anxiety disorders. Some individuals with panic disorder find that even moderately intense exercise can precipitate a panic attack. In this situation it is better to start with low-intensity exercises (such as walking or slow jogging). Depression, so often a co-morbid problem in anxiety disorders, is frequently improved with exposure to sunlight—thus outdoor exercise is often more emotionally beneficial. It doesn't even have to be sunny, just the outdoor light, even on a cloudy day, seems to make people feel better.

In addition to helping anxiety and depression, exercise has many other health benefits. Done regularly, it can reduce your resting heart rate, decrease blood pressure, help to control obesity and diabetes, and reduce stress-related heart disease. A regular exercise program, ideally done on a daily basis, should be part of any plan to treat anxiety disorders.

Focus on Your Sleep

3. Shakespeare wrote "... Sleep that knits up the ravell'd sleeve of care. ..." An adequate amount of good quality sleep is essential for emotional well-being. You simply cannot feel good when you are sleep-deprived. Learn to value your sleep—make it a priority in your life. Stop neglecting your sleep by shortening or interrupting it; if you focus on your sleep and try to obtain adequate rest, it will be much easier to deal with the anxiety problem. Sleep gives you the emotional reserve that you need to cope with any stress, including an emotional disorder. Sleep deprivation (the result of either not enough sleep or poor quality sleep) by itself can make one quite anxious and produce symptoms such as panic disorder.

Practice good sleep hygiene, going to bed at approximately the same time each night (weekends included) and rising at the same time. Most adults need from seven to seven and a half hours of sleep a night. If you are getting over eight hours a night, and still wake unrefreshed, there is something wrong with the quality of your sleep, some reason why that time is not restoring and revitalizing. See your doctor to rule out problems such as sleep apnea, abnormal movements in sleep, restless leg syndrome or a host of other sleep disorders.

Learn a Relaxation Technique

4. Learning a technique to relax is essential to control anxiety, and thus to begin to control your life. In many anxiety disorders the anxiety itself takes control of your physical and mental processes, initiating and then propagating a chain of events that, once begun, you are unable to stop: for example, increased breathing, tingling, dizziness and increased heart rate. Relaxation techniques allow you to take control of your body's functions and thus prevent the anxiety that forces these symptoms to occur. For example, progressive relaxation is a technique in which you focus on tensing and then relaxing one single group of muscles at a time. You might begin with the muscles in your lower legs: tightening and then relaxing them, and then progress to the muscles in your thighs. There are many different relaxation techniques that can help—including biofeedback, breathing retraining (a technique in which the common problem of hyperventilation—breathing unusually deeply or rapidly—is addressed), diaphragmatic breathing—breathing from the stomach—and many others.

Take a yoga class in which you will learn meditation, focusing on a simple body process such as breathing or the production of a simple sound. All of these techniques teach you to control many of your vital physical functions (such as respiration) and calm your mind, thereby enabling you to concentrate on a simple body function—cleaning your mind of the barrage of stresses that accompany everyday life. It is necessary not only to learn the relaxation technique, but also to practice it regularly and faithfully—at least twice a day—so that the technique becomes automatic, part of your daily life, and thus can be called into effect whenever anxiety or stress become a problem.

Get a Complete History and Physical from Your Doctor

5. Anxiety disorders are complex illnesses, with variable manifestations and mechanisms; therefore, it is necessary to get a complete history and physical in order to be certain that there is no medical cause or aggravating factor for your anxiety problem. The list of possible causes is endless; your doctor is trained to diagnose and treat them. In addition, your doctor will look for the complications and associated problems of anxiety disorders (such as hypertension, co-morbid illness or substance abuse), and will help you with these. He or she will also act as coordinator for your treatment, if necessary organizing investigations and psychological treatment—such as cognitive behavioral therapy—and, perhaps, prescribing medications.

Stop Caffeine

6. Caffeine, one of the most commonly used chemicals in our society, can cause any or all of the symptoms of anxiety disorders. We certainly know that excess caffeine can produce anxiety symptoms in everybody, but it is not well known that some people will have anxiety-like symptoms with even

a small dose of caffeine (as little as one cup of coffee a day). Some people, it seems, are simply more susceptible to the effects of the drug. Interestingly, our sensitivity to caffeine increases as we age—you might not be able to tolerate the two or three cups of coffee that you enjoyed when you were twenty. Caffeine is present in coffee, tea, cola drinks (and some non-cola soft drinks), chocolate, cocoa and many medicines (where it is used as a stimulant to counteract the effects of chemicals with a sedative side effect). Also, it is a common component in cold medicines and pain relievers. Even if caffeine is not the cause of your anxiety disorder, it can certainly make it much worse. We know that caffeine will precipitate panic attacks in those prone to the problem, can interfere with sleep, and can make obsessive-compulsive disorder worse. If you are a regular user of caffeine, it is best that you slowly decrease the amount over several days or even weeks; abrupt withdrawal from caffeine can aggravate anxiety symptoms and produce headaches.

Stop Alcohol and Drugs

7. The relationship between anxiety disorders and alcohol (and other drugs) is very complex; they are intimately inter-related. Alcohol abuse is very commonly seen with anxiety disorders (for example, it is seen in 25 percent of those with panic disorder and 18 percent of those with social phobia). Conversely, alcoholics have a much higher incidence of anxiety disorders than the general population. For example, in one study of alcoholics, 32 percent were found to have a diagnosis of social phobia. In many situations it is difficult to determine which problem came first—the alcohol abuse or the anxiety disorder. Alcohol is a sedative; it decreases feelings of awareness and vigilance and thus helps

the symptoms of anxiety. Unfortunately, these symptoms are worse as the alcohol wears off. There seems to be a rebound effect causing increased vigilance and alertness in the brain as the drug is metabolized. This produces a paradox; alcohol is used to treat the symptoms of anxiety, but the alcohol aggravates these symptoms. Alcohol also interferes with sleep, preventing its restorative function and thus reducing your emotional reserve. Abstinence from alcohol has been shown, in many studies, to decrease fear, anxiety and panic-like symptoms. The discontinuation of alcohol is thus essential in treating these problems. However, rapidly discontinuing alcohol use after prolonged, moderate intake can produce a syndrome of hyperalertness, with shakiness, visual hallucinations and extreme anxiety called delirium tremens. Gradual reduction is advisable.

Similarly, drug use (prescription, over-the-counter or street drugs) often complicates anxiety disorders. It is essential to review with your doctor any medical or prescription drugs that you are currently using for other medical problems to ensure that these are not contributing to your anxiety problem. Over-the-counter drugs (drugs available without prescription) should be considered in this list as well, as many of them (such as cold tablets and analgesics) have compounds that can complicate the problem.

Street drug use is very common in those who suffer from anxiety disorders—especially marijuana, which, though it might help to reduce the symptoms of anxiety temporarily, often compounds the difficulties of management and insight. Cocaine use can produce panic disorder that, unfortunately, sometimes persists long after the initial drug use has stopped. Hallucinogenic drugs such as ecstasy and LSD can produce symptoms such as vivid hallucinations, flashbacks and intense sensory stimulation that are identical to post traumatic stress disorder. The use of any street drug complicates an anxiety disorder and interferes with its proper treatment. You cannot get better until these are discontinued.

Family and Friends—How Can You Help?

The families and friends of those suffering with anxiety disorders are often confused and overwhelmed by the incapacity in their loved one. Many of the symptoms and behaviors seem bizarre, irrational and yet intensely powerful. Although you want to reach out and try to help, you are afraid to make the situation worse. You are not sure whether to use "tough love," encouraging your loved one to confront the problem directly or to accommodate yourself and others to the behaviors and anxieties. Many of these disorders are impossible to ignore, and people who have them make excessive and unreasonable demands, disrupting the stability of families and relationships, and affecting the quality of lives around them. Here are some suggestions as to how you can help:

- Learn all you can about the particular disorder. This allows you to understand the nature of the disorder, and to see a pattern in what might seem to be completely random and disconnected thoughts and behaviors. Knowledge of the disorder helps you to understand that treatments are available and quite effective.
- Encourage your loved one to seek professional help. These disorders are, by definition, disabling, and rarely are they able to be treated completely without help. Persuade your loved one to see the family doctor or a psychologist to begin the process. It is not reasonable to expect those affected to solve the problem on their own.

- Be part of the treatment team. Participate (with permission) in the assessment and treatment plans. Be included in the loop.
- Recognize situations that might be more difficult (such as a crowded room in panic disorder). These are times when your support will be needed.
- Recognize that you are not alone in trying to cope with these disorders. Support groups are available (see Resources on page 164), as is information to deal with the disorders. Encourage your loved one to take advantage of this support, and participate in it.
- Be optimistic. These problems, although often severe, are usually quite amenable to treatment.

Recent Developments

The overwhelming result of the rapid increase in knowledge of these disorders is the fact that they are very amenable to treatment. For most people, a combination of learning about the problem, modifying behavior and expectations (through cognitive behavioral therapy), and sometimes the use of medicine can produce a spectacular improvement in the quality of life. For some disorders (such as phobia) simple exposure therapy, limited to only a few sessions, is usually enough to eliminate the problem. For other anxiety disorders (such as obsessive-compulsive disorder) that are more complicated and prolonged in course, the appropriate use of medicine and psychological therapy produces a marked degree of relief as the symptoms are controlled.

It is important to emphasize that these problems need a professional and objective approach. Your doctor will assess the problem and coordinate the various treatments.

Table of Drug Names

Drug Type	Generic Name	Some Common Brand Names
Serotonin reuptake inhibitors	citalopram	Celexa
	fluoxetine	Prozac
	fluvoxamine	Luvox
	paroxetine	Paxil
	sertraline	Zoloft
Tricyclic antidepressants	amitriptyline	Elavil
	clomipramine	Anafranil
	desipramine	Norpramin
	imipramine	Tofranil
Other antidepressants	bupropion	Wellbutrin
	mirtazapine	Remeron
	venlafaxine	Effexor
	moclobemide	Manerix
Tranquilizers and sedatives	alprazolam	Xanax
	buspirone	Buspar
	clonazepam	Rivotril, Klonopin
	diazepam	Valium
	temazepan	Restoril
	lorazepam	Ativan
	zopiclone	Imovane
	oxazepam	Serax

Glossary

Agoraphobia: an intense, irrational fear of open spaces or public places in which escape might be difficult of help unavailable.

Comorbidity: a term used to describe the situation where two or more diseases or disorders occur at the same time in the same person.

Dissociation: a psychiatric term used to describe the separation of mental processes and reactions from conscious awareness. Seen in trauma and panic disorder, dissociation functions as a protective mechanism often experienced as the feeling that one is no longer inside one's own body.

Generalized/Global Anxiety Disorder: an anxiety disorder in which excessive and uncontrolled worrying produces chronic anxiety and symptoms of increased muscle tension, sleep disturbance, fatigue and irritability.

Hyperthyroidism: a medical disorder of the thyroid gland in which excessive amounts of thyroid hormone is released into the blood stream producing symptoms of weight loss, anxiety, tremors, rapid heart beat and sometimes abnormal protrusion of the eyeballs.

Norepinephrine: a hormone produced by the adrenal gland (and some brain cells). It produces increased heart rate, elevated blood pressure and anxiety symptoms.

Obsessive Compulsive Disorder: an anxiety disorder in which obsessions (thoughts and images that repetitively intrude into the patient's thinking and produce anxiety) are coupled with compulsions (physical actions done to reduce the anxiety of the obsession).

Opiod: a synthetic narcotic or any one of a number of naturally occurring chemicals (such as endorphin) that relieve pain.

Panic Attack: an attack of acute, extreme anxiety associated with physical symptoms of shortness of breath, palpitations, dizziness, etc.

Panic Disorder: an anxiety disorder consisting of recurring, disabling panic attacks and often including avoidance behavior such as agoraphobia.

Pheochromocytoma: a rare benign tumor of the adrenal gland that produces increased secretion of the hormones epinephrine and norepinephrine.

Phobia: a persistent, intense and irrational fear of a specific object, activity or situation.

Post Traumatic Stress Disorder: an anxiety disorder that results from severe emotional or physical trauma and results in chronic anxiety, insomnia, flashbacks, intrusive memories, irritability and chronic disability.

Rumination: the mental act of constantly dwelling on certain ideas or problems without progressing to solutions.

Simple Phobia: also known as specific phobia—an irrational fear of a specific object (such as a spider) or situation (such as heights).

Sleep Apnea: a sleep disorder in which severe snoring leads to complete obstruction of the airway with a decrease in blood oxygen levels and repeated awakenings overnight. Sleep apnea is a common cause of chronic tiredness and fatigue. It can be associated with high blood pressure.

Social Anxiety Disorder: a disorder in which individuals experience severe anxiety in social situations where they fear they may be embarrassed or humiliated by contact with others.

Somatization: the process in which mental experiences or stress is converted to physical symptoms.

Tolerance: in drug therapy, the phenomenon wherein the same dose of medicine, used over time, produces less effect.

Trauma: any physical wound or injury. In psychiatry, trauma refers to any distressing or emotionally disturbing experience.

Trichotillomania: the compulsive pulling out of one's hair.

Further Resources

Organizations

U.S.

Obsessive-Compulsive Foundation
676 State Street
New Haven, CT 06511
Tel: (203) 401-2070
Fax: (203) 401-2076
www.ocfoundation.org

Social Phobia/Social Anxiety Association
2058 E. Topeka Drive
Phoenix, AZ 85024
www.socialphobia.org/index.htm

Canada

**Anxiety Disorders Association of Canada/Association
Canadienne des Troubles Anxieux (ADAC/ACTA)**
P. O. Box 461, Station D,
Scarborough ON
M1R 5B8
1-888-223-2252
www.anxietycanada.ca

Canadian Mental Health Association
8 King Street East, Suite 810
Toronto ON M5C 1B5
Tel: (416) 484-7750
Fax: (416) 484-4617
www.cmha.ca

Internet

Anxiety and Panic Site—a search engine for anxiety-related disorders and resources.
www.anxiety-panic.com

Books

Antony, M.M., M.G. Craske and D.H. Barlow. *Mastery of Your Phobia* (client workbook). St. Antonio, TX: The Psychological Corporation, 1995.

Antony, M.M. and R.P. Swinson. *The Shyness & Social Anxiety Workbook*. Oakland, CA: New Harbinger Publications, 2000.

Craske, M.G. and D.H. Barlow. *Mastery of Your Anxiety and Panic,* 3rd ed. (client workbook). Boulder, CO: Graywind Publications, 2000.

Greenberger, D. and C.A. Padesky. *Mind Over Mood: A Cognitive Treatment Manual for Clients*. New York, NY: Guilford Press, 1995.

Index

Note: A page number in italic indicates a figure, table or boxed text.

acrophobia *67*, 70
adolescents
  hairpulling 128
  panic episodes 128
  situational phobias 129
  social anxiety 34
adrenaline (hormonal)
  in normal alarm 14, *15*
  in panic attacks 50
age factors
  blood/injury/injection phobia 75
  caffeine effects 48
  generalized anxiety disorder 23–24
  hoarding 117
  hydrophobia 71
  obsessive–compulsive disorder
    108, 117
  panic disorder 44
  social anxiety disorder 34
agitation 86, 89
agoraphobia
  and quality of life 65, 68–69
  defined *67*, 67–68
  in history *41*
  prevalence 68
  with flight phobia 73
  with panic disorder *41*, *52*, *59*,
    67–68
alarm biology 12–16

alcohol
  causing panic symptoms 56
  importance of reducing and
    stopping 30, 155–56
  withdrawal from *10*
alcohol abuse
  generalized anxiety disorder 27, 31
  obsessive–compulsive disorder 111
  panic disorder 59
  social anxiety disorder 36
alprazolam
  about *149*
  for performance anxiety 37
alternative therapies 140–42
amitriptyline 145
amok *34*
amphetamines *10*
analgesics 56
anger 108
angina *10*, *55*
animal phobia
  about 66–67
  in children 66, 129
antidepressants
  about 144–45
  causing panic symptoms 56
  for generalized anxiety disorder
    30
  for obsessive–compulsive disorder
    220
  for panic disorder 60
  for post traumatic stress disorder
    100

for social anxiety disorder 37
antihistamines 56
anxiety
    abnormal 1–2, 8–9, 16
    and alarm biology 12–16
    caused by drugs *10*, 28, 56, 131
    caused by medical problems *10*,
        28, 131
    defined 7
    in childhood 123
    in post traumatic stress disorder
        89
    positive aspects 1, 8
    signs and symptoms 6–7
anxiety disorders, *see also specific*
    disorders
    causes 10
    coping with 151–59
    costs 1
    education about 152
    in children 5, 23, 44, 71, 73,
        77–78, 108, 112–15, 119–20,
        124–33
    prevalence 1, *4*, 9
    prognosis 134
    recent developments 159
    signs and symptoms 11
    stigma 1
    treatment 134–50
    types 4–5, 9
asthma *10*, 55
astraphobia 70
ataque de nervios *34*
aversion 65–66
avoidance behavior 27–28

benzodiazepines
    about 149–50
    for childhood anxiety disorders
        132
    for generalized anxiety disorder
        30–31
    for needle phobia 75
    for performance anxiety 37
beta blockers 37
blood phobia
    about 67, 73–77, 80, 82
    in children 75, 129

blood pressure changes
    in panic 42
    in phobias 65
blood pressure, high *10*, 55
blood sugar, low *10*
blushing 33
body dysmorphic disorder 118
brain
    anatomy *14, 143*
    and alarm biology 13–14
    focus of drug treatment 142–44
    in obsessive–compulsive disorder
        119
    in post traumatic stress disorder
        95
breathing increase
    in panic 42
    in phobias 65
breathlessness 89
bronchitis 55
bugs, fear of 66–67, 129
buspirone
    about 147
    for generalized anxiety disorder
        30

caffeine
    causing anxiety symptoms *10*
    causing panic symptoms 48, 53,
        56–57
    importance of reducing and
        stopping 30, 155–56
catecholamines
    in normal alarm response 14, *15*
    in post traumatic stress disorder
        97–98
chamomile 140–41
checking, compulsive 115
chemicals *10*
chest tightness 45
children
    causes of anxiety disorders 24,
        125–26
    diagnosis of anxiety disorders
        131
    hairpulling by 127–28
    normal anxiety 123–24
    panic in 44, 128

signs and symptoms of anxiety
disorders 124–25
treatment of anxiety disorders
131–33
with generalized anxiety disorder
23, 130
with obsessive–compulsive
disorder 108, 112–15, 119–20,
127–28, 130–31
with phobias 71, 73, 77–78, 129
with selective mutism 127
with separation anxiety 126
with social anxiety disorder 129
with symmetry obsession 115
choking
in panic attacks 45
"lump in throat" feeling 72
choking phobia 72–73
chorea 119
chronic obstructive pulmonary
disease (COPD) 10
citalopram 146
claustrophobia 69–70, 73
cleanliness obsession 113–14
clinging to parents 124
clomipramine
about 145
for generalized anxiety disorder
30
for obsessive–compulsive
disorder 220
for post traumatic stress disorder
100
clonazepam
about 149
for generalized anxiety disorder
30
cognitive behavioral therapy
about 135–36
behavioral aspects 137–38
cognitive aspects 136–37
effects 138–40
for childhood anxiety disorders
131–32
for generalized anxiety disorder
29–30
for obsessive–compulsive disorder
121
for panic disorder 60

for post traumatic stress disorder
100
for social anxiety disorder 36
combat fatigue 90
complementary therapies 140–42
compulsions
defined 5, 105–6
in children 124
without obsessions 112
concentration problems
in generalized anxiety disorder 20
in panic disorder 42, 46
in post traumatic stress disorder
86, 89
in social anxiety disorder 33
congestive heart failure 10, 55
contamination fear 113–14
COPD (chronic obstructive
pulmonary disease) 10
corticotropin–releasing hormones
98
cortisol
in normal alarm response 15
in post traumatic stress disorder
98
costume phobia 73
coughing 45
cultural factors 34

danger reaction 12–16
death
fear of 42
of parent 125
of spouse 24
debriefing 99–100
decongestants 56
densensitization therapy 75
dental phobia 71
depression
with generalized anxiety disorder
27
with obsessive–compulsive
disorder 111
with panic disorder 58–59
with social anxiety disorder 35
desipramine 145
diabetes 55
diagnosis
anxiety disorders in children 131

generalized anxiety disorder
19, 28
obsessive–compulsive disorder
107
panic attacks 47
panic disorder 54–56
post traumatic stress disorder
86–89
diarrhea 11, 42, 46
diazepam *149*
diet 53–54
disease phobia 72
disgust feelings 108
dissociation 99
divorce
effect on adults 23–24
effect on children 125
dizziness 11, 46
doctor, role 155
doll phobia 73
doubt, obsessive 115
drugs, *see also specific drugs*;
substance abuse; *table on page 161*
causing anxiety symptoms *10*,
28, 131
causing panic symptoms 56
for childhood anxiety disorders
132
for generalized anxiety disorder
30–31
for obsessive–compulsive
disorder 120
for panic disorder 61
for post traumatic stress disorder
100
for social anxiety disorder 37
importance of reducing 157–58
where they work in brain 142–44

eating disorders 111
electroconvulsive therapy 121
employment
generalized anxiety disorder 23
obsessive–compulsive disorder
109
panic disorder 54
performance problems 20
phobias 75

post traumatic stress disorder
91–92, *93*
social anxiety disorder 35
endocrine diseases *55*
endorphins
in normal alarm response 15
in post traumatic stress disorder
98–99
epinephrine (hormonal)
in normal alarm response 14, *15*
in phobias 65
evolution, and phobias 79–80
exercise
to reduce anxiety disorders 30,
152–53
triggering panic attacks 48, 52
exposure therapy
for phobias 81–82
for social anxiety disorder 36
eye movement desensitization and
reprocessing 100, *101*

fainting
evolutionary reason for 76, 80
in anxiety disorders 11
in blood/injury/injection phobia
76–77
in panic attacks 42, 47
family and friends, *see also* genetic
factors
accommodation of person with
anxiety disorder 69, 108–10
role in treatment 59, 121, 158–59
fatigue
chronic 11
in childhood anxiety disorders
124
in generalized anxiety disorder
19–20
fear
defined 7, 64
in childhood 123
in childhood anxiety disorders
124–25
in obsessive–compulsive disorder
108
in phobias 64–66
in post traumatic stress disorder
86

fibromyalgia 11
"fight or flight" response 16, 50, 98
fitness, lack of 20
flashbacks 86–88, 91, 95
flight phobia 73
flooding therapy 81–82
fluoxetine 145–46
flushing 11
fluvoxamine 37
friends *see* family and friends

GAD *see* generalized anxiety
    disorder
gender factors
    generalized anxiety disorder 23
    obsessive–compulsive disorder
        108
    panic disorder 44
generalized anxiety disorder (GAD)
    co–morbidity 26–28, 31
    defined 4, 9
    diagnosis 19, 28
    in children 130
    prevalence 23
    prognosis 26
    signs and symptoms 18–21, 24–26
    treatment 21, 29–31
    who gets it 21–24
genetic factors
    childhood anxiety disorders 125
    generalized anxiety disorder 23
    obsessive–compulsive disorder
        118
    panic disorder 44, 59
    phobias 77
    post traumatic stress disorder
        92–94
globus hystericus 72
glucocorticoids *15*
guilt feelings 97

hairpulling
    in adults 117
    in children 127–28
handwashing compulsion 113
harm thoughts 114–15
headaches
    in anxiety disorders 11

in childhood anxiety disorders
    124
in generalized anxiety disorder
    19
heart problems
    causing anxiety symptoms *10*
    causing panic symptoms *55*
heart rate changes
    in anxiety disorders 11
    in panic attacks 42, 45
    in phobias 64–65
    in post traumatic stress disorder
        89
heights, fear of 67, 70
herbal products
    about 140
    risks 142
    types 140–42
heredity *see* genetic factors
high blood pressure drugs 56
hoarding, compulsive 116–17
homemakers 23
hormones
    and alarm biology 13–15
    and obsessive–compulsive
        disorder 108
    causing anxiety symptoms *10*
    in panic attacks 50
    in phobias 65
    in post traumatic stress disorder
        98
hydrophobia 63, 70–71
hypertension *10*, 55
hyperthyroidism *10*, 55
hyperventilation
    defined 50
    in panic attacks 50, 57
hypervigilance 88
hypoglycemia *10*, 55
hypothyroidism *10*
hysteria 89–90

imipramine
    about 145
    for generalized anxiety disorder
        30
injection phobia
    about 67, 73–77, 80, 82
    in children 129

injury phobia 67, 73–77, 80, 82
injury thoughts 114–15
insomnia *see* sleep problems 11
insomnia, in childhood anxiety
    disorders 124
intrusive thoughts 114–15
irritability
    in generalized anxiety disorder
        20
    in obsessive–compulsive disorder
        108
    in post traumatic stress disorder
        86, 89, 95
irritable bowel syndrome 11

kava 141
koro *34*

life crises, and generalized anxiety
    disorder 24
lithium, for obsessive–compulsive
    disorder 220
lorazepam *149*
    for performance anxiety 37
loss–of–control feeling 151
    in panic attacks 42, 46–47
    in post traumatic stress disorder
        86–87, 98–99
    in social anxiety disorder 33
lung diseases, causing panic
    symptoms 55

MAO inhibitors, for obsessive–
    compulsive disorder 220
marriage, and generalized anxiety
    disorder 23
mask phobia 73
medical conditions
    causing anxiety *10*, 28, 131
    causing anxiety symptoms *10*
medical examination 155
memory loss and changes, in post
    traumatic stress disorder 96, 99
memory problems, in generalized
    anxiety disorder 20
men
    and blood phobia *75*
    and generalized anxiety disorder
        23

and panic disorder 44
and post traumatic stress
    disorder 92, 94
Meniere's disease, causing panic
    symptoms 55
migraine *10*
    causing panic symptoms 55
mitral valve prolapse *10*
moclobemide 149–50
monoamine oxidase inhibitors,
    about 148–49
multiple sclerosis, causing panic
    symptoms 55
muscle ache 11
muscle tension/pain, in generalized
    anxiety disorder 19
mutism, selective 127

nausea 11, 46
needle phobia
    about *67*, 73–77, 80, 82
    in children 129
negative thoughts 136–37
neurological diseases 55
nightmares 86, 95
norepinephrine (hormonal)
    in normal alarm 14, *15*
    in panic attacks 50
    in phobias 65
    in post traumatic stress disorder
        98
numbness
    emotional 86, 88
    physical 45

obsessions
    defined 5, 104–5
    in children 124
    triggers 105
    without compulsions 112
obsessive–compulsive disorder (OCD)
    and perfectionism *109*
    and quality of life 108–10
    causes 118–20
    co–morbidity 111
    cycle 106–7
    defined 5, 9, 104
    diagnosis 107
    in children 130–31

prevalence 108
prognosis 108
signs and symptoms 108–9
treatment 120–21
types 111–18
who gets it 108
with panic disorder 59
OCD *see* obsessive–compulsive
    disorder
out–of–body feeling 42, 46
oxazepam *149*

pain
    abdomen 11, 46, 124
    back 11
    chest 11
    muscles 19
    neck 11, 19
    not felt in acute injury 15
painkillers *56*
pa–leng *34*
panic
    abnormal 41–43
    defined 40
    in children 125, 128
    normal and useful 40–41
panic attacks
    at night *53*, 54
    biological changes during 50–51
    co–morbidity 43, 67–68
    defined 43
    diagnosis 47
    duration 47
    how to help someone having one
        49
    in history *41*
    managing *46*
    prevalence 43
    preventing *46*, *49*, 52–54
    signs and symptoms 45–47, 50
    triggers 48
    who gets them 43–44
panic disorder
    causes 55–56, 59–60
    co–morbidity 27, 58–59
    defined 5, 9, 43
    diagnosis 54–56
    in history *41*
    prevalence 43

prognosis 44
quality of life 52–54
research 56–58
signs and symptoms 42–43
treatment 60–61
who gets it 43–44
with obsessive–compulsive
    disorder 111
paralysis 46
paroxetine
    about 146
    for social anxiety disorder 37
passion flower 141
perfectionism *109*
performance anxiety 33, 37
phenelzine 220
pheochromocytoma *10*, *55*
phobias
    atypical 71–73
    causes 77–80
    common types *67*
    co–morbidity 111
    coping with *75*
    defined 5, 9, 63–64
    dental 71
    in children 124, 129
    prevalence 63
    signs and symptoms 64–66
    situational *41*, *52*, 59, 65, 67–70,
        73, 129
    social *see* social anxiety disorder
    to animals 66–67, 129
    to blood/injury/infection 129
    to blood/injury/injection 67,
        73–77, 80, 82
    to choking 72–73
    to disease 72
    to dolls, costumes, masks 73
    to flight 73
    to nature and environment 63,
        67, 70–71
    to vomiting 73
    treatment *75*, 80–82
post traumatic stress disorder (PTSD)
    and quality of life 88
    causes *90*, 91–93
    co–morbidity 93–94
    defined 5, 9, 85–86
    diagnosis 86–89

historical understanding of
  89–92
prevalence 92, *93*
preventing 99–100
September 11, 2001 87
signs and symptoms 86, 94–95
treatment 100
understanding 94–99
pregnancy
  and herbal medicines 142
  and obsessive–compulsive
    disorder 108
progressive tension therapy *75*
psychological therapy
  for childhood anxiety disorders
    131–32
  for generalized anxiety disorder
    29–30
  for obsessive–compulsive
    disorder 121
  for panic disorder *46*, *49*, 60
  for phobias 81–82
  for post traumatic stress disorder
    99–100, *101*
  for social anxiety disorder 36–37
PTSD *see* post traumatic stress
  disorder

quality of life
  and agoraphobia 65, 68–69
  and obsessive–compulsive
    disorder 108–10
  and panic disorder 52–54
  and post traumatic stress
    disorder 88

rape 89, *90*, 91–92, *93*, 94
reflex, conditioned 78
relaxation therapy
  about 154–55
  for panic disorder *46*, *49*
  for social anxiety disorder 36
religious obsession 117
respiratory problems
  causing anxiety symptoms *10*
  causing panic symptoms *55*
restlessness 11, 19
rituals
  in children 125

in compulsive actions 106
ruminatino 112
running amok *34*

school
  adult limitations 35
  childhood problems 20, 109, 125
secrecy 109
sedatives 56
seizures *10*
selective serotonin reuptake
  inhibitors (SSRIs)
  about 145–47
  for childhood anxiety disorders
    132
  for generalized anxiety disorder
    30
  for obsessive–compulsive disorder
    220
  for panic disorder 60
  for post traumatic stress disorder
    100
  for social anxiety disorder 37
self–esteem, low 33
seniors
  compulsive hoarding 117
  generalized anxiety disorder 23
  panic disorder 44
separation anxiety 126
September 11, 2001 87
serotonin–norepinephrie reuptake
  inhibitors (SNRIs)
  for generalized anxiety disorder
    30
  for obsessive–compulsive disorder
    220
  for post traumatic stress disorder
    100
sertraline
  about 146
  for social anxiety disorder 37
sexual activity
  and anxiety disorder in Asian
    males *34*
  and panic disorder 52
sexual assault 89, *90*, 91–92, *93*, 94
shaking 45
shame 109
shell shock 90

signs and symptoms
  anxiety disorders 11
  anxiety disorders in children
    124–25
  generalized anxiety disorder
    18–21, 24–26
  normal anxiety 6–7
  obsessive–compulsive disorder
    108–9
  panic attacks 45–47, 50
  panic disorder 42–43
  phobias 64–66
  post traumatic stress disorder 86,
    94–95
  social anxiety disorder 32–33
situational phobias
  about 67–70
  in adolescents 129
sleeping pills 56
sleep paralysis *34*
sleep problems
  in generalized anxiety disorder
    20
  in panic disorder *53*, 54
  in post traumatic stress disorder
    86, 89
  reducing 29–30, 153–54
slowness, compulsive 116
smoking cessation products 56
snakes, fear of 66–67, 129
SNRIs *see* serotonin–norepinephrie
  reuptake inhibitors
social anxiety disorder
  co–morbidity 27, 35–36, 111
  defined 5, 9, *67*
  in children 129
  prevalence 34
  signs and symptoms 32–33
  treatment 36–37
  who gets it 34–35
social phobia *see* social anxiety
  disorder
social therapy 36
socioeconomic status 93
sore throat 124
spaces, fear of *see* agoraphobia;
  claustrophobia
SSRIs *see* selective serotonin
  reuptake inhibitors

stammering
  in panic attacks 46
  in social anxiety 33
stereotactic psycho surgery 121
storms, fear of 70
St. John's wort 141–42
streptococcal infection 119–20
stress
  acute reaction to 94–96, 98
  role in childhood anxiety
    disorders 125, 131
  role in obsessive–compulsive
    disorder 108
  role in panic attacks 59–60
stroke 55
stuttering *128*
substance abuse
  importance of reducing and
    stopping 157–58
  with generalized anxiety disorder
    30–31
  with obsessive–compulsive
    disorder 111
  with panic disorder 59
  with social anxiety disorder 36
suicidal thoughts 54
superstition *112*
surgery 121
survivor's guilt 97
sweating
  in anxiety disorders 11
  in panic attacks 42, 45
  in phobias 65
  in social anxiety 33
symmetry obsession 115–16
symptoms *see* signs and symptoms

tantrums 125
temperature fluctuations 45
tension therapy 75
throat, sore 124
thyroid hormone 98
tingling 11, 45
tiredness *see* fatigue
tranquilizers 56
trauma *see* post traumatic stress
  disorder
travel 52, 54

treatment
    about 134–35
    herbal 140–42
    of childhood anxiety disorders
        131–33
    of generalized anxiety disorder
        29–31
    of obsessive–compulsive disorder
        120–21
    of panic disorder 60–61
    of performance anxiety 37
    of phobias 75, 80–82
    of post traumatic stress disorder
        100
    of social anxiety disorder 36–37
    recent developments 159
    role of family and friends 121,
        158–59
    with cognitive behavioral
    therapy 135–40
    with drugs 142–50
trembling
    in panic attacks 45
    in social anxiety 33
trichotillomania
    in adults 117
    in children 127–28
tricyclic antidepressants
    about 144–45
    for generalized anxiety disorder
        30
    for obsessive–compulsive disorder
        220
    for post traumatic stress disorder
        100
tumors *10, 55*

valerian 142
venlafaxine 147–48
vertigo *10, 55*
vomiting
    fear of 73
    in panic attacks 46

war
    and panic disorder *41*
    and post traumatic stress
    disorder 87–91
    and stress reaction 94
    survivor's guilt 97
water, fear of 63, 70–71
weakness 11
withdrawal 109
women
    blood phobia 75
    generalized anxiety disorder 23
    obsessive–compulsive disorder
        108
    panic disorder 44
    post traumatic stress disorder 89,
        91, 92, 93, 94
work *see* employment
worrying
    caused by drugs 28
    caused by medical problems 28
    defined 24
    excessive 25–26
    in generalized anxiety disorder
        18–20, 25–26
    in obsessive–compulsive disorder
        108
    positive aspects 24–25